7-Day Keto

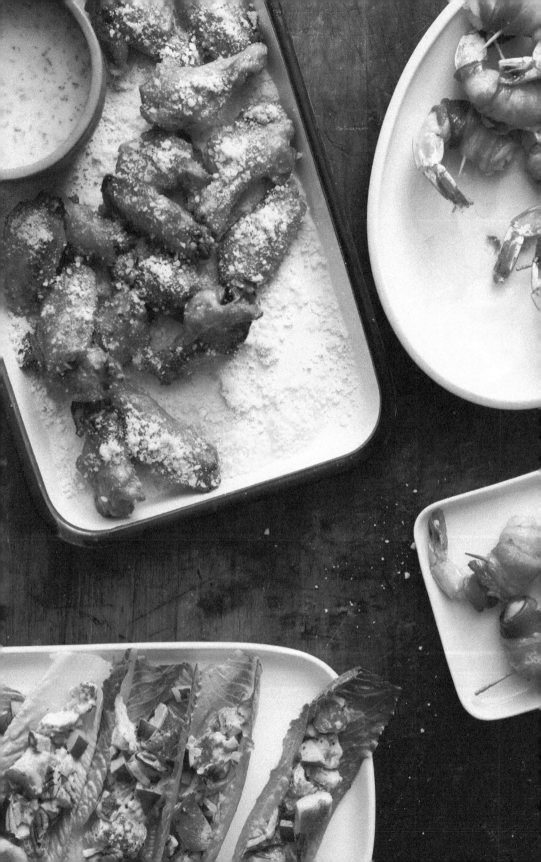

# 7-Day KETO

## THE STARTER GUIDE
### for Ketogenic Diet Beginners

**Mary Alexander**

Photography by Evi Abeler

ROCKRIDGE
PRESS

Interior & Cover Designer: Darren Samuel
Art Producer: Meg Baggott
Editor: Clara Song Lee
Production Editor: Nora Milman

Photography © 2018 Evi Abeler. Food styling by Albane Sharrard.
Author photo by Zack Alexander.

ISBN: Print 978-1-64152-769-9 | eBook 978-1-64152-770-5

R0

*To Kitty,* my sweet mama, my best friend, my "one." I know you're up in heaven, tearing up the dance floor with that big red lipstick smile. We love all the butterflies . . . xox

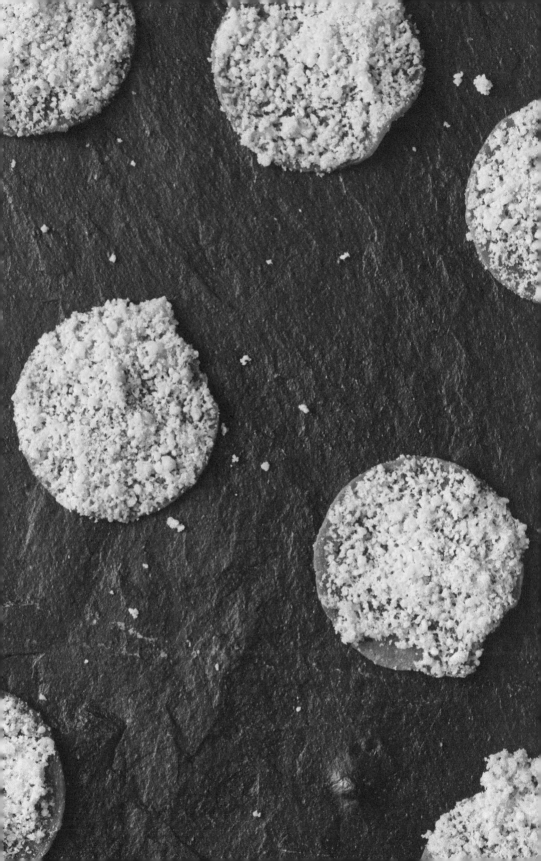

# Contents

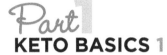
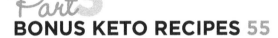
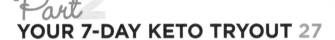

# Introduction

If you had told me five years ago that I'd be writing a lifestyle book on losing weight and getting healthy, I would have laughed. I've spent my entire life struggling to lose weight and have tried every diet out there. Most resulted in losing a few pounds and then gaining back twice as much. I was a binger, and food ruled my life. Like an addict, I used it as my drug of choice to reward and medicate, equally. Lose a pound, eat a cookie. Gain a pound, eat the whole box.

I remember the day I first tipped the scales at over 210 pounds, and I knew my 5' 2" frame couldn't handle any more. It was hard to move. My blood pressure was high, in the first stage of hypertension, and my energy and self-esteem were at an all-time low. I was anxious and couldn't sleep at night—I didn't want to go to the doctor, because I was afraid of what he would tell me. But I knew I had to do something. I began dabbling in low-carb diets and was having success but couldn't maintain the lifestyle. Something was missing.

Then I read about the keto diet. As a low-carb fan, I was intrigued by the significant results others were having, as well as the variety of delicious, real foods they were enjoying, and I was eager to try it. My partner, David, and I decided to start keto. I made a promise to myself that this time I would see it through. I've kept that promise and never looked back. With keto, I was able to eat more than I've eaten on any other diet, and I never got bored with the choices. I stuck with it and got stronger and stronger. With this low-carb, high-fat lifestyle, I've lost over 60 pounds. I no longer "take orders" from food and have gotten binging under control. I maintain a healthy weight and have enjoyed a multitude of health benefits like more energy, less anxiety, a healthy blood pressure, and so much more. Now I welcome going to the doctor and seeing perfect blood panels and other indicators of how healthy I am.

So how does keto work? Your body prefers glucose/sugar from carbohydrates as its primary fuel source. When you take away the carbs, your body turns to burning its own fat stores for fuel instead. This fat-burning mode is known as ketosis, a metabolic state that converts fatty acids into ketones, which are like rocket fuel for your body. In this state of ketosis, glucose levels are lower, creating fewer cravings and sugar crashes, making it a more relaxed lifestyle to maintain over the long haul. The best part is that many of the foods you already enjoy are keto friendly.

In this book, you'll learn the science, the myths, and the rules—that is, which foods to enjoy and which to avoid. Then we'll put together a shopping list and meal plan so you can try the keto diet for seven days. With the foods you bring home and seasonings you probably already have on hand, you'll be able to create delicious and affordable keto-friendly meals and snacks. We'll also put together some simple, five-ingredient recipes that you can use every day.

Like any change, the shift to a keto diet takes a little adjustment. I'll share some treats and tips to get you through it. Ultimately, I think it's much harder to be unhealthy than it is to adjust to this new lifestyle. So, I challenge you to "choose your hard." By choosing health over the status quo, you're setting the groundwork for a more vibrant future. Join me, and we'll explore it together for a week. If you're like me, you'll never look back.

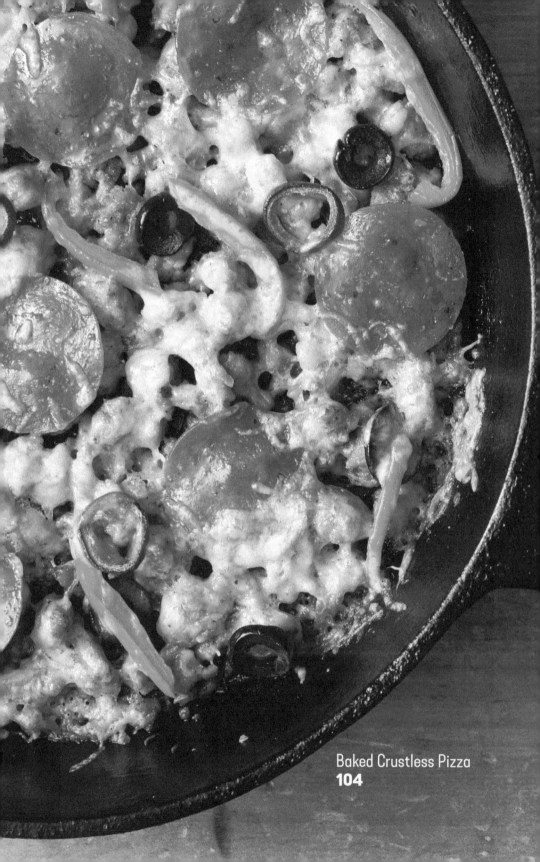

# KETO
# BASICS

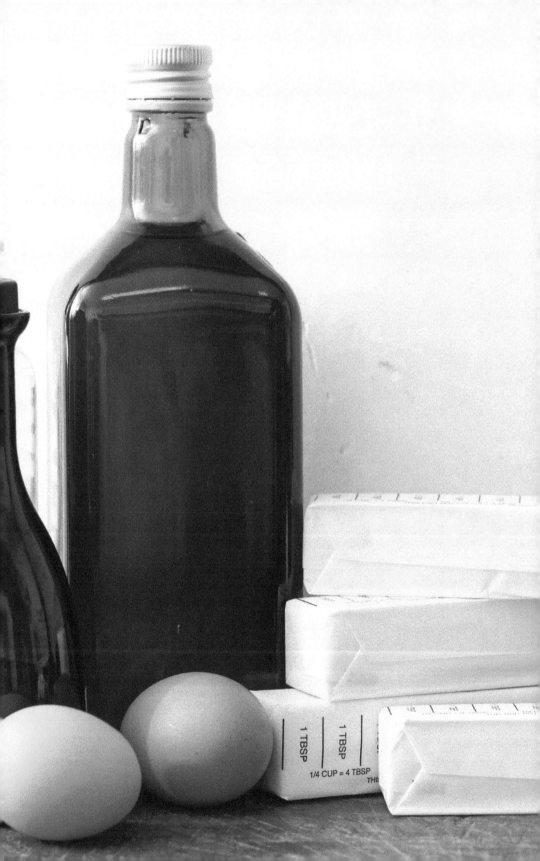

# One
## HOW THE KETO DIET WORKS

In this chapter, we'll cover all the essentials you need to know to begin the keto diet, the science behind it, and its place in a sea of diet choices. We'll also dispel some myths surrounding this diet so you can be fully and accurately informed.

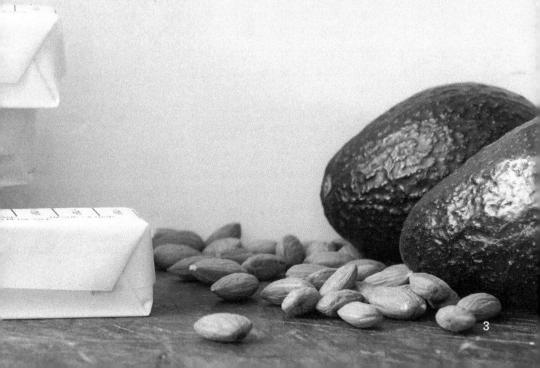

# A MEDICAL DIET GOES MAINSTREAM

Today, many people know someone who's following the ketogenic diet, a low-carb, high-fat diet that causes the body to burn fat instead of carbs for fuel. This lifestyle has gained mainstream attention as a result of social media, but it was originally developed by the medical community to treat epilepsy.

In 1921, Dr. Russell Wilder of the Mayo Clinic proposed a treatment for epilepsy that mimicked the effects of fasting. Researchers in the early 20th century had noticed the way fasting forced the body to burn fat instead of carbs. This change in the body's metabolism reduced the number of seizures in epileptic patients. By eating a diet higher in fat and dramatically lower in carbohydrates, Dr. Wilder's patients entered a similar metabolic state called "ketosis," a process in which the body converts fat into chemicals called ketones and burns ketones instead of its preferred fuel of sugar or glucose.

Since then, the rising popularity of low-carb diets has pushed the ketogenic diet into the spotlight. In the 1970s, Dr. Robert Atkins introduced the concept of ketosis to the general public as part of his Atkins diet. The Atkins diet is similar to keto, except that on Atkins, you eat more protein and gradually increase your carb intake as you get closer to your weight goal, which eventually puts you out of ketosis and stops your body from burning fat. The keto diet grew further in popularity in the mid-2010s, when a growing number of celebrities introduced its benefits to their followers, who posted about the diet on platforms such as Reddit and Instagram. Keto would go on to be the most-googled diet of 2018, despite the fact that it was a century old!

## Treating Health Conditions with Keto

The rapid weight-loss benefits of keto probably get the most attention, but there's also much research connecting it to the successful treatment of other disorders, including epilepsy, diabetes, polycystic ovary syndrome (PCOS), certain forms of cancer, Alzheimer's, and more.

In the United States alone, 1 out of 10 Americans suffers from diabetes, and 90 to 95 percent of those folks are type 2 diabetics. Studies have shown that some diabetics using the ketogenic diet

 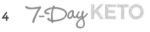

have enjoyed improved glycemic control, and some were able to reduce or discontinue diabetes medications altogether. Because the ketogenic diet can improve insulin sensitivity, it is being researched as a promising treatment for other metabolic conditions like pre-diabetes and obesity.

Polycystic ovary syndrome (PCOS) is the most common endocrine disorder affecting women. Insulin resistance is one symptom, which can make losing weight difficult, and infertility is another. Cleveland Clinic researchers led a study on combatting insulin resistance using a closely monitored keto diet and saw favorable results in achieving weight loss as well as regulating periods and conceiving without ovulation induction.

The keto diet has further been shown to reduce and restrict tumor growth in certain types of cancer. It achieves this by lowering glucose levels in the body, which takes away a fuel source from cancer cells, making it harder for them to survive. Research has also shown that following the keto diet in conjunction with cancer treatment may significantly enhance the success of chemotherapy and radiation treatments.

Although it was initially analyzed for its benefits to epilepsy patients, the ketogenic diet is now being studied to treat other neurological conditions. Research is finding promising results in improving memory and slowing the progression of nerve-related disorders like Parkinson's and Alzheimer's diseases.

## KETO AS A LONG-TERM LIFESTYLE

Currently, there is no research that proves the ketogenic diet is dangerous to follow in the long term. The most common criticism is that the diet's restrictive nature puts followers at risk of missing out on vital nutrients. However, if you're diligent about eating a wide variety of low-carb veggies along with nuts, seeds, and different sources of protein, you can certainly still meet all of your nutritional needs.

How easy it will be to stay on the keto diet depends on you. If you find that the keto diet helps you lose weight and control symptoms and risk factors for health conditions like type 2 diabetes and heart disease, then you might feel very motivated to stick to the diet. Likewise, if you aren't big on carbs to begin with, you might also find the keto diet a good fit. To a great degree, success with any diet depends on your ability to find a variety of foods you like. When I started keto in 2016, it was hard to find premade keto-friendly snacks and food items. However, I was experiencing such wonderful results and unexpected benefits from keto, I didn't mind the extra cooking and quickly learned to make my own keto treats.

Fortunately, the rising popularity of the keto diet has made it much easier to find all kinds of delicious keto-friendly snack items, premade baked goods, cereals, bread, pastas, chips, and more, both at grocery stores and through online retailers. Every year, the booming market of keto products makes it easier for keto dieters to stay on track. Ordering at restaurants is also not nearly as challenging as it used to be, and many restaurants are willing to accommodate diners who request low-carb modifications to their dishes.

## MAKING THE KETO DIET WORK

We've discussed how the keto diet works by making the body burn fat instead of sugar/glucose to achieve a metabolic state of ketosis. Specifically, the way we do this is by cutting out refined grains and sugar, such as bread, pasta, pastries, flour, rice, sweet desserts, and cereal, and replacing them with high-fat, low-carb foods like fatty meats and fish, eggs, low-carb vegetables, nuts, seeds, and natural fats like olive oil and butter.

### Understanding Macros

You'll hear the word "macros" used a lot when talking keto. Macro-nutrients, or macros, give you energy and are the basic building blocks of your diet. The three macronutrients are carbohydrates, proteins, and fats, whose energy can be quantified by this equation: carbs + protein + fat = total calories. Depending on your individual goals, macros can be tracked as percentages of the food you eat every day. Each person's target macros may be different, so you'll want to figure out your individual macro needs. To do this, you can go online and search "macro calculators." There are many available free of charge (see the Resources section, page 126). You'll be able to enter information such as your height, weight, and gender, and they'll calculate optimal macros for whatever goals you have.

When you first start the keto diet, you'll want 70 to 75 percent of your daily calories to come from fat, 20 to 25 percent to come from protein, and 5 to 10 percent to come from carbs. An easy way to keep up with this is by getting a diet app to use on your phone. There are many to choose from, and for the most part, free of charge. I use MyPlate. You input the foods throughout the day, and it tallies up your calories and macros as you go along.

If you don't want to track macros in the beginning, you can set a daily goal to stay under 20 net carbs (total carbs - fiber - sugar alcohols = net carbs). We'll discuss net carbs in further detail in chapter 2.

### Getting into Ketosis

"Getting into ketosis" is the process of making your body burn fat instead of sugar/glucose. Getting into and staying in ketosis is the initial goal with keto, and the best way to get there is by restricting your carbohydrates and upping your fat intake. To reach ketosis and start burning fat, your body must first burn through all of its stored glucose/sugar. That process can take as little as two to four days or sometimes longer.

Some great signs that you're in ketosis are that you're losing weight or your appetite feels like it's gone. Some weird but equally great signs of ketosis are that you have a funky, fruity taste in your mouth or that your breath is horrible in general—welcome to ketosis. Some people may experience short-term symptoms such as nausea or feeling run-down, even sick. This is often called the "keto flu." These symptoms tend to be mild and are usually caused by the loss of water weight and electrolytes in the first few days. Many folks give up at this point, but if you can stick it out, you'll find that the keto flu doesn't last long. Push past the symptoms by replacing those lost electrolytes with supplements. Drink more water, sugar-free electrolyte sports drinks, pickle juice, or my favorite, warm bone broth.

There are three ways you can scientifically test whether you're in ketosis: checking for ketones in your urine or blood, or checking for acetone in your breath. In the beginning, you can use ketone-testing strips for urine. It's not mandatory, but it can help you make sure you're on track. These over-the-counter strips measure the ketones that spill over into a person's urine—something that happens when the body is not used to processing ketones efficiently. Once you've been in ketosis for a while and your body begins to use ketones more efficiently, you might consider testing with a ketone and glucose meter, which offers the most accurate results by testing your blood. I use the Keto-Mojo. The final way to check ketones is by measuring acetone in your breath. There are several breath ketone meters on the market as well. The Ketonix Acetone Breathalyzer is pricey but has great reviews.

# COMMON CONCERNS AND MYTHS

There are a lot of concerns and myths about the ketogenic diet. Here are a few of the most common ones:

**You can't eat fruit on keto.** This is untrue. Many fruits are high in sugar, but strawberries, blackberries, raspberries, and blueberries are all keto friendly and great in moderation with a meal or as a snack.

**It's too hard to give up bread and sweets.** This really varies from person to person. Today, with all the keto-friendly goodies and recipes available, many people are discovering that it's easier to give up bread and sweets than they thought it would be.

**You can't ever cheat on keto.** It's true that if you cheat on keto, there's a good chance of getting thrown out of ketosis; because of this, most people think twice before cheating. But I like to remind my followers that they're also free to come back to keto after cheating, too. Each meal is a fresh chance to get back into keto and feel good about choosing your health over your cravings again.

**It's impossible to travel and eat out on keto.** I have found this to be quite untrue. The keto diet may feel a little more challenging when you're traveling, but it's definitely not impossible. Most places you visit will have the keto basics (meats, cheese, olives, eggs, and more) at any market. Many restaurants have low-carb menu items readily available, and even if you don't see them on the menu, you can usually request modifications to a dish that make the meal keto-friendly. To learn more, see "What If You Want to Eat Out?" on page 38.

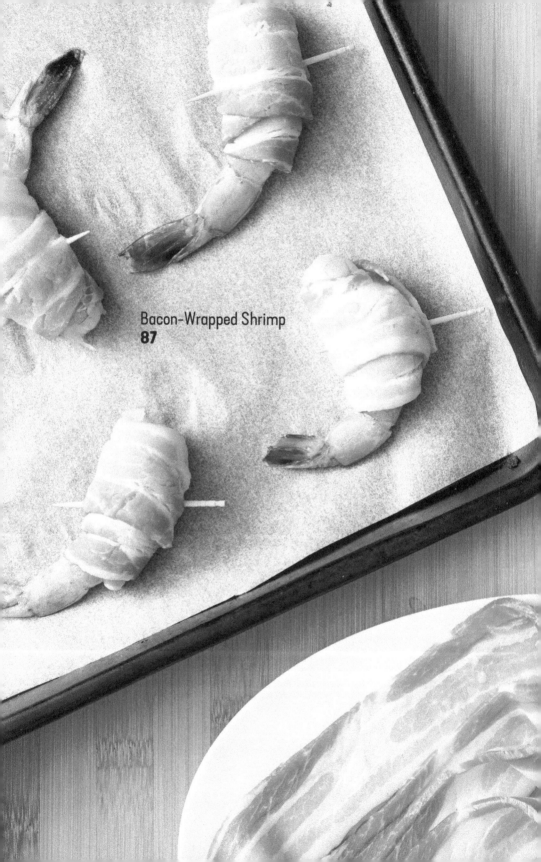

Bacon-Wrapped Shrimp
**87**

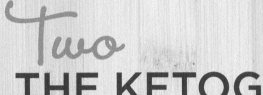

# Two
# THE KETOGENIC DIET RULES

In this chapter, we'll explore the rules of eating keto. You'll learn the hows and whys of keto living, especially as it pertains to the goal of getting 70 percent of your calories from fat, 20 percent from protein, and 10 percent from carbohydrates. I'll also throw in some special tips and tricks that will make the job easier.

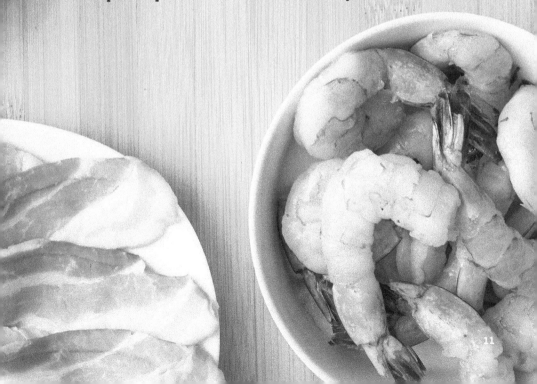

# EAT MOSTLY FAT

The keto diet operates by restricting carbohydrates and encouraging consumption of high amounts of fat. The goal is to reach a state of ketosis, where your body burns fat for energy due to the lack of carbohydrates. To achieve this, you'll want to set a daily goal that 70 to 75 percent of your calories come from fat.

The easiest way to reach your daily goal is to incorporate foods into your diet that have macros of 75 percent fat or higher. Some keto-friendly (and tasty) things you're probably already eating, along with their fat percentages, are:

**BUTTER, 100%**

**MAYONNAISE, 100%**

**HEAVY WHIPPING CREAM, 95%**

**SOUR CREAM, 93%**

**RANCH DRESSING, 93%**

**MACADAMIA NUTS, 90%**

**CREAM CHEESE, 87%**

**BACON, 85%**

**PORK SAUSAGE, 80%**

**EGG YOLKS, 79%**

**SALMON, 76%**

**AVOCADOS, 75%**

 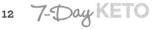

In 1950, physiologist Dr. Ancel Keys hypothesized that saturated fat caused cardiovascular heart disease and should be avoided. In many studies since, this hypothesis has been debunked. Some fats are healthier than others, but whether it's unsaturated fats found in foods like avocados, nuts, and olive oils, or saturated fats found in foods like butter, red meat, and eggs, they're all beneficial in some way.

There are some unhealthy fat sources to stay away from, including processed trans fats and vegetable oils (oils extracted from seeds), such as corn, canola, grapeseed, peanut, soybean, and sunflower oils, margarine, and vegetable shortening.

## MODERATE PROTEIN INTAKE

A protein balance is important. Generally, your goal in keto is to keep protein around 20 to 25 percent of your total calories. The body converts excess protein into glucose, a process called gluconeogenesis, which can potentially kick you out of ketosis. However, protein does a great job of keeping you full, so you don't want to eat too little, either. If you find yourself getting hungry, a little protein will usually do the trick.

Unlike fats and carbs, protein isn't stored in the body, so it's important to get enough protein every day. Protein is essential for strong bones and building a healthy immune system. A protein deficiency can cause hair loss, skin problems, nail issues, and even result in muscle loss, as well as put you at an increased risk of illness.

Generally, I would recommend following the guideline of getting 20 to 25 percent of your daily calories from protein, but people react differently to protein. If you eat more than that and you're having an issue staying in ketosis, simply drop back a little. The important thing is to make sure you always get enough protein.

A great way to stay in balance with fat and protein is to eat fattier cuts of meat. Some good choices include a beef ribeye or New York strip steak, chicken thighs, pork ribs, and hamburger meat—all easily ordered in a restaurant or thrown on the grill at home. Lean meats like skinless chicken, turkey, beef, and pork that have been trimmed of fat are fine as well, but you'll need to compensate with fat elsewhere to meet your goal.

# RESTRICT CARBOHYDRATES

You've learned that to reach ketosis and start burning fat as fuel, you must dramatically restrict your carb intake. Everyone is different, but generally, you should be eating around 30 to 50 carbs per day, which will work out to around 5 to 10 percent of your calories. Some people may be able to eat additional carbs and stay in ketosis, while others might need to cut back.

Keto is a pretty restrictive lifestyle with regard to carbs, and some people find it easier to start out by staying under 20 net carbs per day instead of tracking macros or percentages. I did this in the beginning, and it worked well for me. For the first few months, I aimed for 20 net carbs daily, and anything that fit in that calculation was fair game. I was able to lose 15 pounds quickly, and during that time I became very familiar with the different carb counts on food items and how they affected my ability to reach and stay in ketosis. When my weight loss began to slow down and stall, I started tracking macros. It was a smooth transition, and I began to lose weight once again.

## Net Carbs

You can track either total carbs or net carbs. Total carbs mean all the carbs that a serving of food contains. Net carbs are the actual carbs absorbed by the body that have an impact on your blood sugar. To calculate the net carbs of a whole food, such as a piece of fruit, we take the total amount of carbs minus fiber. For example, an avocado has 16 grams of carbs and 12 grams of fiber. So, 16 - 12 = 4 net carbs. Fiber doesn't get used in the body because it doesn't break down, so it can be deducted.

## Sugar Alcohols

Sugar alcohols are man-made sweeteners used in many low-carb goodies, and we'll use some of them in recipes in this book. Examples are erythritol, maltitol, sorbitol, and xylitol. Some can be substituted directly for sugar, and some are much sweeter. Sugar alcohols operate a lot like fiber in that they don't get used in the body because they don't break down, so they can also be deducted to determine net carbs. The equation is carbs - fiber - sugar alcohols = net carbs.

 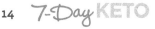

Not all sugar alcohols are created equal, however, and not everyone can achieve and stay in ketosis while eating them. There are the lucky few who can down any goody with sugar alcohols and see no effect on their level of ketosis, and others who can eat the same thing and get thrown out. It's simply a trial-and-error process.

## HYDRATE, HYDRATE, HYDRATE

Dehydration is a common side effect of ketosis. Your body is used to eating carbs and storing that energy as glycogen (the stored form of glucose). When you restrict carbs and burn through all your stored glucose, you lose a great deal of water weight and electrolytes in the process. High levels of ketones can also cause frequent urination, further contributing to the loss of water and electrolytes.

When starting a keto diet, this loss of water weight and electrolytes can make you feel run-down and nauseated, something described earlier as the keto flu. It's crucial from the very start, and throughout ketosis, to always stay hydrated; otherwise, you may experience headaches, muscle cramps and spasms, weakness, fatigue, and more.

The simple way to treat and avoid dehydration is by drinking more water, electrolyte supplements, sugar-free electrolyte sports drinks, pickle juice, bone broth, and consuming more liquids in general.

# BULLETPROOF COFFEE

Bulletproof coffee, BPC for short, is a delicious, high-fat, high-calorie concoction that's used to enhance energy and endurance before a workout. The original recipe came from Dave Asprey, the creator of the Bulletproof Diet. It also serves as a substitute for breakfast or a quick "pick-me-up" throughout the day. BPC is made with 8 to 12 ounces of freshly brewed coffee, 1 to 2 tablespoons of unsalted butter, whipping cream or half-and-half, and 1 to 2 tablespoons of medium-chain triglyceride (MCT) coconut oil or powder. MCT oil can be a little hard on your stomach, so some people prefer the powder. Some people also add collagen powder, artificial sweeteners, unsweetened cocoa, or other sugar-free flavors. I like to add Perfect Keto's MCT oil powder and their collagen powder to mine. You can use a frother or blender to turn BPC into a creamy latte, or simply stir it up. BPC is considered great for keto, as the high-fat butter keeps you satiated and full for hours, while the MCT oil or powder provides quick, clean energy and aids in appetite suppression—all via hot, caffein-ated coffee.

# WHAT ABOUT INTERMITTENT FASTING?

Intermittent fasting involves eating within a window of 8 hours and fasting for the remaining 16, a method that can provide benefits in the keto lifestyle. A sample eating window for someone doing intermittent fasting might start with the first meal of the day at 11:00 a.m. and end with the final meal of the day eight hours later at 7:00 p.m. The rest of the day, from after your last meal at 7:00 p.m. until your first meal the next day at 11:00 a.m., is spent fasting. Some people shorten their eating windows to between four and six hours, but eight is fine.

When combined, keto and intermittent fasting yield outstanding results. Keto mimics fasting in that it forces the body to burn fat for energy when starved of carbohydrates. Intermittent fasting sets the body up to efficiently burn fat between meals by lowering insulin, which can be very helpful to reach and/or stay in ketosis or achieve more aggressive weight-loss results.

The eight-hour eating window can be altered to fit any schedule, but it's best to eat earlier in the day and not snack at all, especially at night, although you'll want to stay hydrated at all times. Studies have shown that eating early and fasting at night also helps with metabolism. It's not for everyone and certainly not mandatory—just another method worth considering as you explore the keto lifestyle.

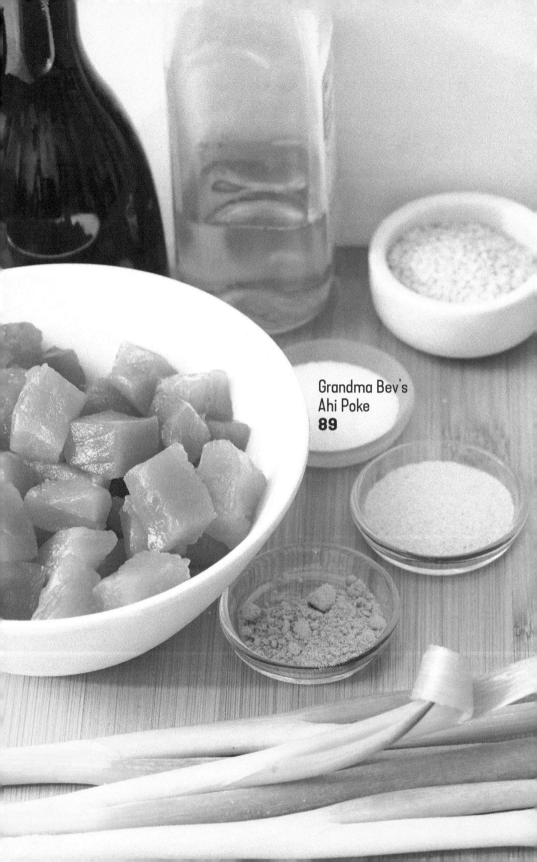

Grandma Bev's
Ahi Poke
**89**

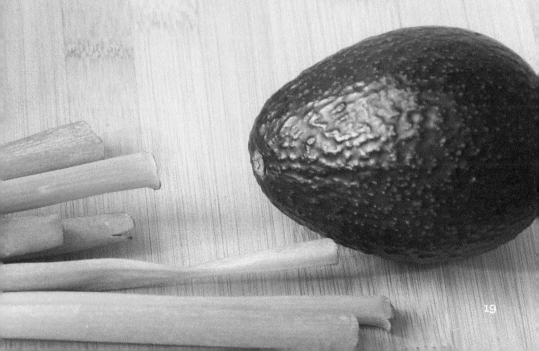

# *Three*
# WHAT TO EAT ON THE KETO DIET

Now that you understand how the body works with regard to keto, let's explore the food! We'll walk through what a clean keto diet consists of and what foods to eat, limit, and avoid. I'll also answer some frequently asked questions and talk about a few special keto ingredients.

## CLEAN VERSUS "DIRTY" KETO

The keto diet originated for the purpose of healing the body, with a focus on nutrient-rich whole foods that are naturally higher in fat and lower in carbs. This book loosely follows the "clean" version of keto, which is the healthiest way to get into ketosis and burn fat instead of carbs. There's also another version—"dirty" keto—which can do the same thing. So, what's the difference?

Clean keto focuses on eating high-quality whole foods that are minimally processed or preserved to achieve ketosis. Grass-fed beef, free-range eggs, and organic vegetables are staples of a clean keto diet, and I encourage using them whenever possible, as your budget allows. On the other hand, followers of dirty keto can eat whatever they want to reach ketosis, so long as they maintain macro percentages of 70 to 75 percent fat, 20 to 25 percent protein, and 5 to 10 percent carbs. Processed foods are allowed in dirty keto, as are foods from favorite fast-food restaurants. Keto-friendly versions of foods like cookies, cakes, and chips are also fine on a dirty keto diet.

For people new to the ketogenic lifestyle, the dirty keto diet can be a real lifesaver, making a daunting diet feel a lot more achievable because you don't have to rely on cooking every single meal. Many people have had great success following the keto diet while still eating at some of their favorite restaurants and taking the edge off their cravings with keto-friendly snacks.

However, over time, the dirty keto diet can turn on some people. By continuing to eat keto-friendly versions of cookies and chips, they never break the habit of eating junk food. Additives like antibiotics, pesticides, and preservatives can slow down the body's healing process. Plus, many people find that the processed ingredients in keto-friendly snacks, like sugar alcohols and chemicals, start to have a negative effect on their bodies and even kick them out of ketosis.

As in all good things, moderation is key. In the beginning, dirty keto isn't bad and can make the transition to a low-carb diet much easier; whatever works for you is fine. But in the long run, a successful ketogenic lifestyle is all about an escalation: making good, better, and then the best choices. For many people, following the clean keto diet most of the time, with occasional indulgences in dirty keto meals, seems to work best.

**Foods to Enjoy Freely, Eat in Moderation, or Avoid**

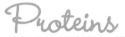

## Proteins

### Enjoy Freely
Bacon, beef, chicken, clams, cod, deli meats, eggs, flounder, ham, herring, hot dogs, lobster, oysters, pepperoni, pork, pork belly, pork rinds, prosciutto, salami, salmon, sardines, sausage, shrimp, sole, tilapia, tuna, turkey, veal

### Avoid
Breaded meats, deli meats and hot dogs with added sugars, glazed ham, imitation crab meat

## Dairy

### Enjoy Freely
Butter, cream cheese, ghee, halloumi/bread cheese, hard cheeses, heavy cream, mascarpone, soft cheeses, sour cream, string cheese

### Eat in Moderation
Cottage cheese (½ cup), plain Greek yogurt (½ cup)

### Avoid
Condensed milk, custards, milk, puddings, sweet milk, yogurt

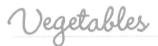

## Vegetables

### Enjoy Freely
Asparagus, cabbage, celery, chives, cucumbers, eggplant, green chiles, kale, leafy greens, lettuce, mushrooms, pickles, radishes, spinach, zucchini

### Eat in Moderation
Artichokes (1 medium), bell peppers (½ cup sliced), broccoli (1 cup), Brussels sprouts (1 cup), cauliflower (1 cup), green beans (1 cup), jalapeños (½ cup sliced), okra (1 cup)

### Avoid

Carrots, corn, parsnips, peas, potatoes, sweet pickles, sweet potatoes, yams

## Fruits

### Enjoy Freely

Lemons, limes, olives, unsweetened coconut

### Eat in Moderation

Avocados (½), blackberries (½ cup), blueberries (¼ cup), raspberries (¼ cup), strawberries (½ cup), tomatoes (3 slices)

### Avoid

Apples, bananas, canned fruits, dried fruits, fruit juices, mangos, oranges, peaches, pears, pineapples

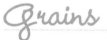

## Grains

### Avoid

Barley, bread, brown rice, cookies, corn tortillas, crackers, flour tortillas, oatmeal, pasta, quinoa, white rice

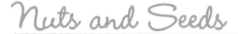

## Nuts and Seeds

### Enjoy Freely

Chia seeds, flaxseed, hemp seeds, sesame seeds

### Eat in Moderation

Almond butter (2 tablespoons), almonds (1 ounce), Brazil nuts (1 ounce), hazelnuts (1 ounce), macadamia nuts (1 ounce), peanuts (1 ounce), pecans (1 ounce), pili nuts (1 ounce), pumpkin seeds (1 ounce), raw peanut butter (2 tablespoons), sunflower seeds (½ cup), walnuts (1 ounce)

### Avoid

Cashews, honey-roasted or glazed nuts, nut butters with added sugars, pine nuts, pistachios

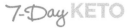

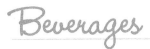

# Beverages

### *Enjoy Freely*
Bone broth, bouillon, coffee, seltzer or sparkling water, tea, unsweetened nut milks, water

### *Eat in Moderation*
Sugar-free sodas (occasionally), sugar-free sports drinks (occasionally)

### *Avoid*
Fruit juices, sodas, sweetened tea

The foods included in the "Enjoy Freely" category can be enjoyed without any limits or moderation. Foods in the "Eat in Moderation" category are keto friendly but often very easy to overeat, and the carbs can add up quickly. It's a good idea to portion out these items so you don't accidentally consume too much. If weight loss slows down or stalls, work to cut back on these. Even if a food is on the list, check labels whenever possible for added sugars. The "Avoid" category lists foods that must be cut completely from the keto diet.

## A WORD ABOUT SPECIAL KETO INGREDIENTS

The marketplace has exploded with keto products, supplements, and ingredients like MCT oil, exogenous ketones, low-carb bread, keto-friendly cookies, chips, and more. I find that many of these are expensive, hard to find, and unnecessary, but if you find some that make staying keto more enjoyable, go for it! The main objective is getting started and staying on track. The longer you follow this lifestyle, the easier it will become.

That said, there are a few special ingredients that are great to have on hand for use in recipes. Note that items you prepare at home will also be healthier versions of the dishes you buy premade or from a restaurant. Most grocers carry these ingredients, but they're also available online. You'll see these ingredients used throughout the recipes in this book.

**FLOUR SUBSTITUTES.** Most keto recipes call for almond flour, but I prefer coconut flour, which has fewer carbs in the equivalent amount of flour and is usually less expensive. We'll use both.

**SUGAR SUBSTITUTES.** Sugar substitutes containing erythritol, xylitol, monkfruit, or stevia are good choices. The two brands I use the most are Lakanto (monkfruit-based) and Swerve (an erythritol blend). Both are available in granular and powdered versions and can be substituted 1:1 for sugar, so they're easy substitutes in traditional recipes. Either one of these brands will be great for recipes in this book and pretty easy to find. Liquid sweeteners are perfect for coffee and drinks. I like stevia and just use the store brands.

**PORK RINDS.** This great low-carb snack also doubles as a flavorful add-in to many dishes and as a replacement for bread crumbs. You'll find them in many fun flavors and brands at grocers and online. My favorite brands are Southern Recipe Small Batch and Pork King Good.

## FREQUENTLY ASKED QUESTIONS

*Do I need to restrict calories on keto?*
Calories always matter in the end, especially if your goal is weight loss, but with keto, eating fewer calories occurs naturally. One of the most significant benefits of keto eating is appetite suppression. By eating greater amounts of fat and moderate amounts of protein, you stay satiated for longer, which allows you to eat fewer calories overall.

*How much weight can I lose on keto, and how long will it take?*
Weight loss is different for everyone. Much of your success will depend on how much weight you have to lose and how closely you follow the guidelines. That said, keto is known for stimulating rapid weight loss. A significant amount of water weight, 10 pounds or more, can be lost in the first few days or couple of weeks, and even more over the first month. After that, the losses continue but depend on your own individual journey.

### Do I need any special supplements for keto?

Electrolyte supplementation (sodium, potassium, magnesium) is essential on keto because you've restricted carbohydrates, which are responsible for water retention. You can make up for the loss by adding supplements, by drinking more liquids, sugar-free sports drinks with electrolytes, and bone broth, and by eating a variety of healthy whole foods. Exogenous ketones, MCT oil, and other supplements are not necessary for keto success.

### Can you drink alcohol on keto?

The short answer is yes. Although sugary cocktails like piña coladas and margaritas are out, an occasional low-carb beer or glass of white wine (reds are a little higher in carbs) is okay. Liquors such as vodka, whiskey, tequila, rum, and others are typically carb-free (as long as they are not flavored—check labels) and are great with sugar-free mixers or over ice. The body burns through alcohol before anything else, so while it might not kick you out of ketosis, it could slow down weight loss. Also, with the lack of carbs in your body, alcohol affects you very quickly, so be cautious about how much you're drinking.

### Do sugar alcohols kick you out of ketosis or slow weight loss?

Different sugar alcohols have varying effects on different people. Some people can eat prepackaged cookies, cakes, and other goodies and experience no issues, while others eat the smallest amounts and get kicked right out of ketosis. When I first started keto, I ate them all the time, but then my weight began to stall, and I really cut back. I've also found it's easier to stay in ketosis using sugar alcohols in my home recipes instead of eating prepackaged treats—it's much less expensive, as well.

### How long does it take to go full keto?

Once you get through the first week of the diet and past the keto flu, if one occurs, your appetite will be suppressed and you'll start feeling the benefits of ketosis. Within a couple of weeks, most people are much more familiar with what foods to eat and what to order in restaurants and are able to prepare a variety of keto-friendly meals and snacks. Just keep it simple, make it fun, and lean into it. Pretty soon, it will become a lifestyle.

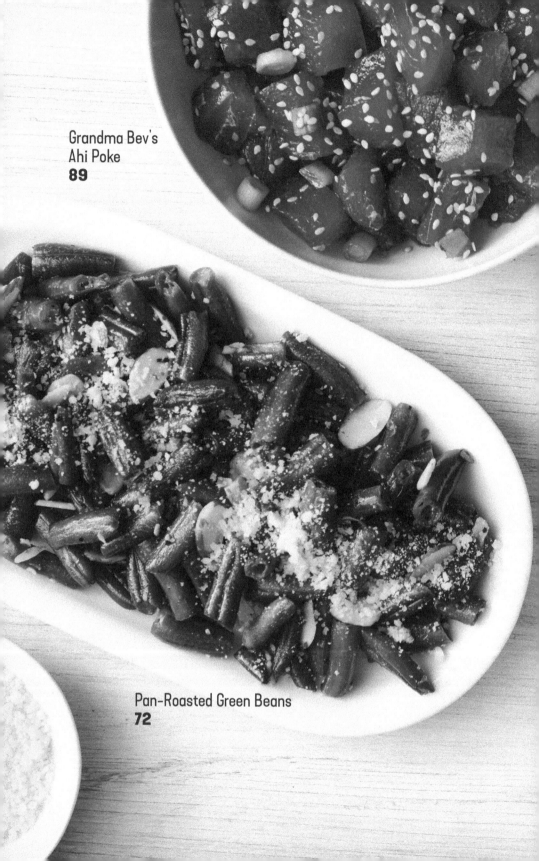

Grandma Bev's
Ahi Poke
**89**

Pan-Roasted Green Beans
**72**

# YOUR
# 7-DAY
# KETO
# TRYOUT

Parmesan Pepperoni Chips
**53**

# Four
# THE 7-DAY MEAL PLAN

Welcome to my keto meal plan! This 7-day plan uses only easy-to-find, everyday ingredients, and several of the recipes contain five* ingredients or fewer for a low-risk, low-pressure intro to keto. Note that these recipes are developed for one person, so if you're doing this plan with someone you live with, you'll want to double the recipes. (*Ingredients that don't count toward the five include salt, pepper, water, oil, and lemon juice.)

# WHAT TO EXPECT (AND NOT EXPECT)

You can expect the first week of keto to be exciting. If you've followed other diet plans, you'll find that keto is nothing like them. Delicious meals and snacks are full of fat, leaving you satisfied and full. Cravings diminish and your appetite becomes suppressed.

### Minor Challenges

Along with being pleasantly full, you may also feel a bit nauseated or run-down, or experience flu-like symptoms after the first two or three days. This keto flu is a sign of dehydration and a good indicator that you're headed toward ketosis. Ease these temporary symptoms by drinking more fluids and supplementing with electrolytes, sugar-free sports drinks, pickle juice, or warm bone broth.

### Major Awesomeness

The awesome part about the first week is that once your body gets through the initial few days, you begin to feel great. Your body enters ketosis by burning through all its stored sugar/glucose and begins burning fat instead. Signs of ketosis include suppressed appetite and a funky, fruity taste in your mouth or bad breath in general—okay, not really awesome, but nothing a little mouthwash won't help. And it means you're on your way! You'll probably also see some dramatic weight loss on the scale with all the water loss, and chances are, you'll begin sleeping better at night and enjoy improved mental clarity throughout the day, along with greater energy.

# HOW TO USE THIS PLAN

This 7-day meal plan is a delicious outline for your first week on the keto diet. The meal plan goes from Monday to Sunday, including three meals a day and one snack. I've kept each day under 20 total carbs, so there's room for additional helpings or snacks if you need to tame some cravings.

All the recipes are "comfort foods" that are meant to be enjoyed, making this first week a fun and easy way to test out the keto lifestyle. The day before you begin, you'll want to prepare the recipes for the

 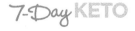

week. I've included a shopping list to help you simplify your meal prep. The recipes I've chosen are simple ones, many with fewer than five ingredients. The ingredients are all inexpensive everyday grocery items, and you will likely already have some on hand in your kitchen.

The plan is flexible, too. If you look at the chart and decide you don't like Buttery Boiled Eggs for breakfast and would rather have two Pancake Muffins instead, go for it. Or if you don't need the snack, cool! The meal plan is simply a suggestion to keep you on track. Many additions and substitutions allow you to make a recipe your own. I've listed carb counts at the bottom of each recipe, so you can follow the plan in its entirety or veer off and do your own thing. Just be sure to check the carb count and serving size for any substitutions or additions, and tally those up at the end of the day to make sure you've stayed under 20 net carbs—at least for the first week.

This is the keto diet, not the "no-fun diet," and with all the delicious, fatty ingredients, I think you'll be more than pleasantly surprised. Yes, you may have some weak moments when you miss the carbs, but I've got more than a few recipes and tricks up my sleeve to get you past that, and it gets easier as you go along. You can do this—*we* can do this!

## 7-DAY MEAL PLAN AND SHOPPING LIST

This meal plan is designed to make starting the keto diet as simple as possible. I tried to select recipes that would feel satisfying and rely on familiar ingredients.

Important note: The meals and snacks in the following chart are meant to correspond to the serving sizes listed in each recipe. For example, the serving size listed in Mary's Chicken Salad on Romaine Boats is three boats, so that is the intended portion in this plan. Any alterations in the serving size will change the number of carbs and other macro numbers, so you'll need to calculate that if you eat a larger or smaller serving.

# Monday 19.5 CARBS • 11.5 NET CARBS

### Breakfast
Pancake Muffin (page 42) and Buttery Boiled Eggs (page 44)

### Lunch
Mary's Chicken Salad on Romaine Boats (page 48)

### Dinner
Bacon Cheeseburger Casserole (page 50)

### Snack
Creamy Deviled Eggs (page 46)

# Tuesday 19 CARBS • 14 NET CARBS

### Breakfast
Cheesy Sausage & Egg Muffin (page 43)

### Lunch
Spicy Creamy Chicken Soup (page 47)

### Dinner
Taco Salad (page 52)

### Snack
Parmesan Pepperoni Chips (page 53)

# Wednesday 19.5 CARBS • 11.5 NET CARBS

### Breakfast
Leftover Pancake Muffin and Leftover Buttery Boiled Eggs

### Lunch
Leftover Mary's Chicken Salad on Romaine Boats

### Dinner
Leftover Bacon Cheeseburger Casserole

*Snack*

Leftover Creamy Deviled Eggs

# Thursday 19 CARBS • 14 NET CARBS

*Breakfast*

Leftover Cheesy Sausage & Egg Muffin

*Lunch*

Leftover Spicy Creamy Chicken Soup

*Dinner*

Leftover Taco Salad

*Snack*

Leftover Parmesan Pepperoni Chips

# Friday 19.5 CARBS • 11.5 NET CARBS

*Breakfast*

Leftover Pancake Muffin and Leftover Buttery Boiled Eggs

*Lunch*

Leftover Mary's Chicken Salad on Romaine Boats

*Dinner*

Leftover Bacon Cheeseburger Casserole

*Snack*

Leftover Creamy Deviled Eggs

# Saturday 19 CARBS • 14 NET CARBS

*Breakfast*

Leftover Cheesy Sausage & Egg Muffin

*Lunch*

Leftover Spicy Creamy Chicken Soup

*Dinner*

Leftover Taco Salad

*Snack*

Leftover Parmesan Pepperoni Chips

# Sunday 19.5 CARBS • 11.5 NET CARBS

*Breakfast*

Leftover Pancake Muffin and Leftover Buttery Boiled Eggs

*Lunch*

Leftover Mary's Chicken Salad on Romaine Boats

*Dinner*

Leftover Bacon Cheeseburger Casserole

*Snack*

Leftover Creamy Deviled Eggs

## Shopping List

You'll want to look through the following shopping list before setting out for the grocery store. You may find that many of these items are already in your pantry and refrigerator.

# Canned and Bottled Items

- ○ Chicken broth or chicken bone broth, 2 (32-ounce) cartons
- ○ Coconut milk, ¼ cup
- ○ Diced tomatoes and green chilies, 3 (10-ounce) cans
- ○ Maple syrup, sugar-free (choose the lowest-net-carb version)
- ○ Mayonnaise, ¾ cup
- ○ Ranch dressing, 2 cups
- ○ Salsa, small jar (look for the lowest-carb version)
- ○ Yellow mustard

# Dairy and Eggs

- ○ Butter, 16 tablespoons (2 sticks)
- ○ Cheddar cheese, grated, 39 ounces (approximately 5 cups)
- ○ Cream cheese, 3 (8-ounce) bricks
- ○ Eggs, large (35)
- ○ Heavy whipping cream, 1 cup
- ○ Parmesan cheese, finely grated, ½ cup
- ○ Sour cream, ¼ cup

# Meat

- ○ Bacon, 6 slices

- ○ Breakfast sausage, 4 ounces

- ○ Chicken, 8 (12.5-ounce) cans or 3½ pounds cooked and chopped or store-bought rotisserie chicken

- ○ Ground beef, 75% lean, 4 pounds

- ○ Pepperoni slices, 6-ounce bag

# Pantry Items

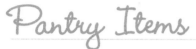

- ○ Baking soda

- ○ Black pepper, freshly ground

- ○ Chili powder

- ○ Cinnamon

- ○ Coconut flour, small bag

- ○ Cumin

- ○ Garlic powder

- ○ Garlic salt

- ○ Paprika

- ○ Sea salt

- ○ Seasoned salt

- ○ Vanilla extract

# Produce

- ○ Red onion, small (1)

- ○ Romaine lettuce leaves, whole (15)

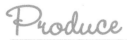

# MARY'S PREFERRED BRANDS

The following products are ones I've come to choose based on their carb count, flavor, and/or overall quality. Try these or find your own favorites:

*Bone/chicken broth*
Kettle & Fire

*Butter*
Kerrygold Unsalted

*Canned green beans*
Allens Italian Cut Green Beans

*Coconut flour*
Bob's Red Mill Organic Coconut Flour

*Coconut milk*
Thai Kitchen Organic

*Cottage cheese*
Kalona (organic, least amount of carbs, but hard to find)

*Creole seasoning*
Tony Chachere's Original Creole Seasoning

*Deli meat*
Oscar Mayer Deli Fresh

*Diced tomatoes and green chilies*
Ro-Tel

*Low-carb tortillas*
Cutdacarb (online only); La Banderita Carb Counter Wraps

*Mayonnaise*
Hellmann's

*Parmesan cheese (shaker bottle)*
Kraft

**Parmesan crisps (store-bought)**
Whisps

**Pepperoni slices**
Hormel Original

**Pork rinds**
Southern Recipe Small Batch and Pork King Good

**Ranch dressing**
Original Hidden Valley Ranch

**Salsa**
Mateo's

**Sea salt**
Redmond

**Seasoned salt**
Lawry's

**Sugar-free brown sugar**
Swerve

**Sugar-free confectioners' sugar**
Lakanto Powdered Monkfruit with Erythritol

**Sugar-free granulated sugar**
Lakanto Monkfruit with Erythritol (Golden)

**Sugar-free maple syrup**
Cary's

## WHAT IF YOU WANT TO EAT OUT?

Inevitably, there will be times that you need to—or want to—eat out, either during this 7-day keto tryout or sometime in the future. Don't be intimidated into thinking that you won't be able to stay on track. Eating out on keto is pretty easy. When it comes to restaurants, any fast-food or sit-down place with a hamburger on the menu is your best bet, especially when you're first starting out. Simply order the

 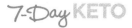

burger you'd like with no bun or as a salad. You might also ask for the sauce to be put on the side. And go for the toppings—there's nothing better than a big half-pound patty on a bed of lettuce with cheese, crispy bacon, sliced avocado, and maybe even a fried egg!

Mexican restaurants are also very easy. You can order fajitas without the tortillas or even request the dish as a salad with grated cheese, sliced avocado, and sour cream as the dressing. You could also ask for ranch dressing, but a lot of restaurants make their own, and homemade versions may contain more carbs than you'd think.

What about pizza? This may be one of my faves! Pick the all-meat pizza with cheese and no sauce and ask them to bake all the ingredients—without the crust. It retains all of the great pizza flavor, and the chef will usually go out of their way to make it look very appealing.

When I'm not sure about a restaurant's offerings, I'll go online earlier in the day and peruse the menu to determine what my best options would be. When I get to the restaurant, there's no stress, and I just order what I know will be delicious and keep me on track.

When you visit restaurants, don't be afraid to ask for what you want. Many are well prepared to offer special low-carb/keto options and more than happy to accommodate your wishes. Have fun with it—eating out is great, and you can still do it in style!

## ABOUT THE RECIPES

Many of the recipes will use no more than five ingredients, not counting salt, pepper, oil, water, or lemon juice. Every recipe in the book will contain a tip for variations, substitutions, or other helpful information. Each recipe also contains nutritional information, including macros, even though you don't need to track them for the 7-day plan—I've tracked them for you!

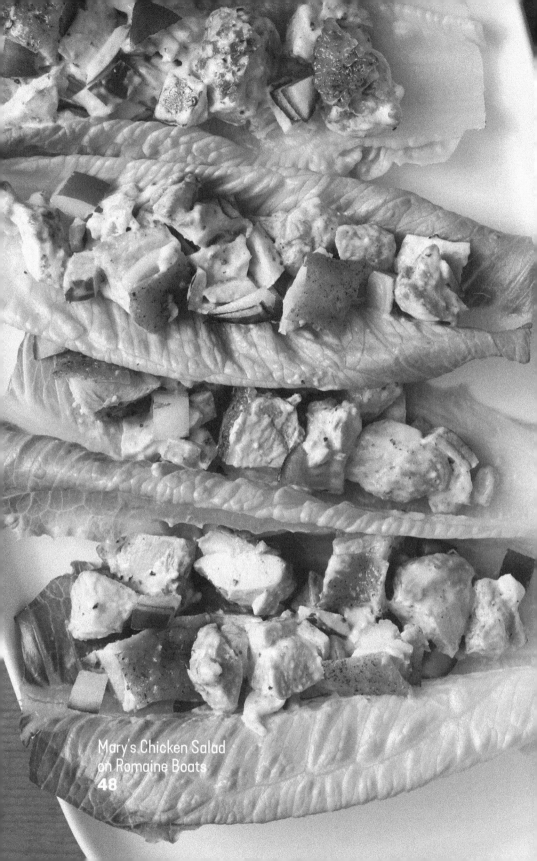

Mary's Chicken Salad
on Romaine Boats
48

# Five
# MEAL PLAN RECIPES

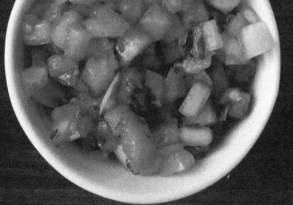

# Pancake Muffins

**PREP TIME:** 10 minutes / Cook time: 15 minutes

When it comes to breakfast food, pancakes are at the top of my list, so having one that's not only keto friendly but also made for a grab-and-go meal, hot or cold, is total greatness! Feel free to use any nut milk in place of the coconut milk.

Nonstick cooking spray (optional)

¼ cup coconut flour

½ teaspoon cinnamon

⅛ teaspoon baking soda

Pinch sea salt

3 large eggs

¼ cup coconut milk

2 tablespoons sugar-free maple syrup

¼ teaspoon vanilla extract

6 tablespoons (¾ stick) butter, for serving

1. Preheat the oven to 350°F. Prepare a 6-cup muffin pan with cooking spray or cupcake liners and set aside.

2. In a small bowl, mix together the coconut flour, cinnamon, baking soda, and salt.

3. In a medium bowl, whip together the eggs, coconut milk, syrup, and vanilla until fluffy.

4. Pour the flour mixture into the egg mixture and mix until just incorporated. The batter will be lumpy.

5. Divide the mixture evenly between the prepared muffin cups.

6. Bake for 15 minutes.

7. Let rest a few minutes and then top each muffin with ½ tablespoon of butter.

**TIP:** Customize your muffins with sugar-free chocolate chips, blueberries, pecans, cooked breakfast sausage—whatever! Just be sure to add the additional carbs to your total. These also freeze beautifully, so go ahead and double the recipe if you'd like extra.

---

**Per Serving (1 muffin)** Calories: 208; Total fat: 17g; Carbohydrates: 8.5g; Fiber: 6g; Protein: 5g; Net carbs: 2.5g

 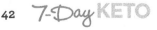

# Cheesy Sausage & Egg Muffins

**12 MUFFINS**

**PREP TIME:** 10 minutes / Cook time: 30 minutes

There's nothing better for breakfast than eggs, but sometimes it's fun to shake things up, and these Cheesy Sausage & Egg Muffins really do the trick. Eggs get elevated with savory sausage and a pair of tasty cheeses, all baked up in convenient muffin tins for a mess-free breakfast on the run.

Nonstick cooking spray (optional)

8 large eggs

6 ounces cream cheese

2 tablespoons butter

½ teaspoon freshly ground black pepper

½ teaspoon garlic powder

4 ounces cooked breakfast sausage

½ cup grated Cheddar cheese

1. Preheat the oven to 350°F. Prepare a 12-cup muffin pan with cooking spray or cupcake liners and set aside.

2. In a blender or with a hand mixer, mix the eggs, cream cheese, butter, pepper, and garlic powder until fluffy.

3. Divide the mixture evenly between the prepared muffin cups.

4. Sprinkle each cup evenly with the sausage and cheese.

5. Bake for 30 minutes. Serve warm.

**TIP:** Get creative—you can substitute or add diced tomatoes, green chiles, onion, peppers, bacon, ham, any flavor cheese—the list goes on. These muffins are also great topped with hot sauce or salsa. Hot or cold, they're always a winner! Just be sure to add any additional carbs to your total.

---

**Per Serving (1 muffin)** Calories: 168; Total fat: 15g; Carbohydrates: 1g; Fiber: 0g; Protein: 7g; Net carbs: 1g

# Buttery Boiled Eggs

**PREP TIME:** 5 minutes / Cook time: 25 minutes

Hard-boiled eggs are a staple in my refrigerator. They fill a multitude of wonderful snack and meal options. If you keep some on hand, this chopped twist on the hard-boiled egg will deliver up a warm and buttery breakfast in about 2 minutes. They are absolutely delicious!

**12 large eggs, at room temperature**

**2 tablespoons butter (see step 6)**

**½ teaspoon sea salt**

**½ teaspoon freshly ground black pepper**

1. Place the eggs in a large pot. Add enough cold water to cover the eggs by a couple of inches.

2. Slowly bring the eggs to a boil over medium-high heat.

3. Once the water begins to boil, remove the pot from the stove and cover.

4. After 15 minutes, transfer the eggs to a bowl of ice-cold water to cool.

5. Peel 3 eggs, place them in a bowl, and slice them up. Place the butter on top and sprinkle with the salt and pepper. Microwave for 30 to 40 seconds, mix, and enjoy.

6. Each time you prepare 3 eggs for a meal, repeat step 5 with the butter, salt, and pepper.

**TIP:** Store remaining eggs, peeled or unpeeled, in the refrigerator. If peeled, refrigerate in a resealable bag. Although these Buttery Boiled Eggs are my favorite just the way they are, you could also add cooked breakfast sausage or bacon, grated cheese, cream cheese, sour cream, and so much more. Just be sure to add the additional carbs to your total.

---

**Per Serving (3 eggs)** Calories: 265; Total fat: 21g; Carbohydrates: 1g; Fiber: 0g; Protein: 19g; Net carbs: 1g

# Creamy Deviled Eggs

**6 SERVINGS**

**PREP TIME:** 15 minutes

It seems like deviled eggs only show up at the holidays, but they're really a great snack and perfect to serve or share on any occasion. There are so many versions available, but these extra-creamy ones are my fave! Directions for hard-boiling eggs are included in the Buttery Boiled Eggs recipe on page 44 (steps 1 to 4).

**6 large hard-boiled eggs**

**¼ cup mayonnaise**

**1 tablespoon cream cheese, at room temperature**

**1 teaspoon yellow mustard**

**⅛ teaspoon garlic salt**

**¼ teaspoon freshly ground black pepper**

**1 teaspoon paprika, for garnish**

1. Peel the eggs and dry them with paper towels.

2. Cut each egg in half lengthwise, and gently transfer the yolks into a bowl. Set aside the egg whites.

3. With a fork, mash all the yolks until ground up. Add the mayonnaise, cream cheese, mustard, garlic salt, and pepper. Mix vigorously until the mixture is creamy.

4. Using a piping bag, a resealable bag with a cut-off corner, or a spoon, fill each egg white half generously with the yolk mixture. Sprinkle each egg with paprika. Store covered in the refrigerator.

**TIP:** If you love deviled eggs, go ahead and make some extra. They're a perfect keto-friendly snack and so easy to tote along on the go. Instead of paprika, try sprinkling them with bagel seasoning, or even place a slice of bacon on top. The possibilities are as endless as your imagination.

**Per Serving (2 deviled eggs)** Calories: 136; Total fat: 11g; Carbohydrates: 1g; Fiber: 0g; Protein: 6.5g; Net carbs: 1g

# Spicy Creamy Chicken Soup

15 SERVINGS

**PREP TIME:** 10 minutes / Cook time: 30 minutes

Loaded with chicken and tasty flavors, this soup is a favorite at our house. Yes, it makes a lot and the recipe is easy to cut in half, but believe me, it goes fast. And because it's so keto friendly, you're liable to want two bowls instead of one!

2 (32-ounce) cartons chicken broth or bone broth

1 (8-ounce) brick cream cheese, cubed

4 (12.5-ounce) cans chicken or 1¾ pounds chopped cooked boneless skinless chicken breasts or rotisserie chicken

2 (10-ounce) cans diced tomatoes and green chilies, undrained

½ cup ranch dressing

½ cup heavy cream

1 teaspoon garlic powder

1 teaspoon sea salt

1 teaspoon freshly ground black pepper

15 ounces grated Cheddar cheese

1. In a stockpot over medium heat, combine the broth, cream cheese, chicken, tomatoes and green chilies, ranch dressing, heavy cream, garlic powder, salt, and pepper.

2. Simmer for 30 minutes, stirring occasionally.

3. Portion into individual bowls and sprinkle each with ¼ cup of Cheddar cheese. Enjoy!

**TIP:** Other goodies you can add to boost the flavor even more include fresh green chiles, cilantro, lime juice, peppers, bacon, jalapeños, any variety of grated cheese, or a dollop of sour cream on top. Just be sure to add the additional carbs to your total.

**Per Serving (8-ounce cup)** Calories: 383; Total fat: 27g; Carbohydrates: 7g; Fiber: 0g; Protein: 27g; Net carbs: 7g

# Mary's Chicken Salad on Romaine Boats

**4 SERVINGS**

**PREP TIME:** 10 minutes

Chicken salad is a wonderful energy-boosting staple to have in your refrigerator. Whether you snag a bite on the way out the door or class it up on a romaine boat, this flavorful chicken salad will awaken your taste buds and keep you energized. Feel free to use a store-bought rotisserie chicken or one you make yourself, too.

4 (12.5-ounce) cans chicken, drained, or 1¾ pounds chopped cooked boneless skinless chicken breasts or rotisserie chicken

¼ cup chopped red onion

1 teaspoon seasoned salt

1 teaspoon freshly ground black pepper

1 teaspoon garlic powder

½ cup mayonnaise

¼ cup sour cream

12 whole romaine lettuce leaves

¾ cup ranch dressing

1. In a large bowl, add the chicken. Use a fork to break apart the bigger chunks.

2. Add the red onion, seasoned salt, pepper, and garlic powder, and toss to thoroughly mix.

3. Add the mayonnaise and sour cream, and mix well. If the mixture seems dry, add a little more sour cream and mayonnaise. This will not affect the carb count.

4. On a plate, lay down three romaine leaves. Spread ¼ cup of chicken salad down the center of each leaf. Stack the extra romaine leaves inside a gallon-size resealable bag with a paper towel and store in the refrigerator until ready to use.

5. Drizzle 1 tablespoon of ranch dressing down the center of each chicken salad boat.

**TIP:** Chicken salad is so versatile—give it a boost with chopped pecans, grated cheese, bacon bits, salsa, Sarayo Sauce, or other condiments or add-ins. Just be sure to add the additional carbs to your total. Store the remaining chicken salad in a resealable container or covered bowl in the refrigerator. If it dries out overnight, simply add some more sour cream or mayonnaise.

---

**Per serving (3 boats with ¼ cup chicken salad in each)** Calories: 576; Total fat: 36g; Carbohydrates: 6g; Fiber: 2g; Protein: 57g; Net carbs: 4g

# Bacon Cheeseburger Casserole

**PREP TIME:** 30 minutes / Cook time: 30 minutes

Is there any better comfort food than a big, fat, juicy bacon cheese-burger? This casserole is easier and tastes even better the next day. This recipe makes 10 servings, so feel free to cut the recipe in half, but it won't go to waste, especially if you make it on a chilly, cozy football day.

3 pounds
ground beef

1 (8-ounce)
brick cream
cheese, cubed

1 (10-ounce) can
diced tomatoes
and green
chilies, drained

6 large eggs

½ cup heavy cream

1 teaspoon
freshly ground
black pepper

1 teaspoon
seasoned salt

1 teaspoon
garlic powder

1 cup grated
Cheddar cheese

6 slices crispy
cooked bacon,
crumbled

Yellow mustard,
for garnish

1. Preheat the oven to 350°F.

2. In a skillet over medium heat, brown the beef, breaking it apart with a wooden spoon. Once it has fully browned, drain completely.

3. Add the cubed cream cheese to the skillet with the meat, mixing well to combine.

4. Add the tomatoes and green chilies to the skillet, stirring well.

5. Pour the meat mixture into a 9-by-13-inch casserole dish and spread evenly.

6. In a separate bowl, whip together the eggs, heavy cream, pepper, seasoned salt, and garlic powder.

7. Pour the egg mixture over the top of the meat in the casserole dish.

8. Sprinkle the cheese over the top of the casserole, and top with the crumbled bacon. Bake for 30 minutes.

9. Let the casserole sit for 10 to 15 minutes. Drizzle yellow mustard across the top and serve.

TIP: Try adding in some fresh green chiles, sugar-free ketchup, mayonnaise, or salsa instead of mustard. Just be sure to add the additional carbs to your total.

---

**Per Serving (1/10 of casserole)** Calories: 675; Total fat: 58g; Carbohydrates: 3g; Fiber: 0g; Protein: 34g; Net carbs: 3g

# Taco Salad

**3 SERVINGS**

**PREP TIME:** 10 minutes / Cook time: 10 minutes

Taco Salad is such a classic, fast, and well-loved meal. Everyone in my family has their own quirky little ways of making it, but for the most part, the basic recipe is the same and full of Tex-Mex flavor. In this recipe, we'll make enough taco meat for three salads, but for future ease, you may want to keep a container on hand at all times!

1 pound ground beef (I use 75 percent lean)

¼ cup salsa

1 teaspoon ground cumin

1 teaspoon chili powder

3 whole romaine lettuce leaves, chopped into bite-size pieces

1½ cups grated Cheddar cheese

6 tablespoons ranch dressing

1. In a skillet over medium heat, brown the meat, breaking it up with a wooden spoon. Once it has browned, drain well.

2. Add the salsa, cumin, and chili powder to the meat, and mix well.

3. In a large salad bowl, add a third of the chopped lettuce. Store the extra lettuce in the refrigerator inside a gallon-size resealable bag with a paper towel.

4. Add one-third of the taco meat to the top of the salad along with ½ cup of grated cheese and 2 tablespoons of ranch dressing. Toss well and devour!

**TIP:** This recipe is the simplest version of a dish you can take in countless directions. Add some chopped avocado, bacon bits, chopped tomatoes, sour cream, pico de gallo, etc. Just be sure to add the additional carbs to your total. Store the remaining taco meat in a resealable container or covered bowl in the refrigerator.

---

**Per Serving (1 salad)** Calories: 852; Total fat: 72g; Carbohydrates: 11g; Fiber: 5g; Protein: 41g; Net carbs: 6g

# Parmesan Pepperoni Chips

**PREP TIME:** 5 minutes / Cook time: 15 minutes

I'm a "chip and dipper" at heart, so one of the things I really missed when I started keto was chips. I found pepperoni slices early in the game, and that was pretty good, but when I discovered Parmesan Pepperoni Chips—wow, what a crispy snack!

1 (6-ounce) bag
sliced pepperoni

½ cup finely grated
Parmesan cheese

1. Preheat the oven to 425°F. Line a baking sheet with parchment paper.

2. Lay each pepperoni slice down on the parchment paper, trying not to overlap.

3. Bake for 10 minutes, remove from the oven, and with a paper towel, dot each pepperoni slice to soak up the grease.

4. Immediately shake enough Parmesan cheese over all the pepperoni slices to lightly cover them.

5. Return the baking sheet to the oven and bake for another 3 to 4 minutes, until the pepperoni slices look crispy.

6. Remove from the oven and transfer the slices from the baking sheet to paper towels. Store leftovers in an airtight bag for up to 2 days in the refrigerator. Reheat in the oven to bring back their crispness.

**TIP:** These little chips are great for dipping in ranch or blue cheese dressing or some guac, too. Just be sure to add the additional carbs to your total.

**Per Serving (about 14 chips)** Calories 174; Total fat: 15g; Carbohydrates: 0g; Fiber: 0g; Protein: 10g; Net carbs: 0g

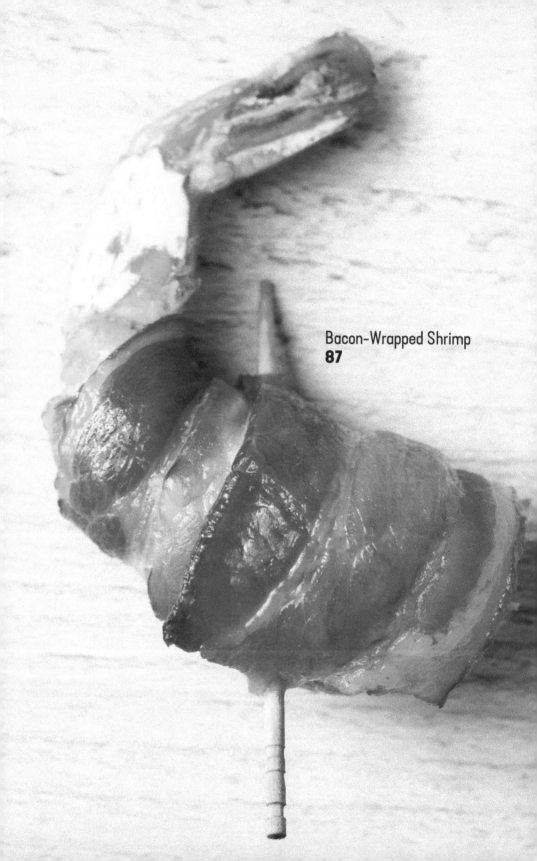

Bacon-Wrapped Shrimp
**87**

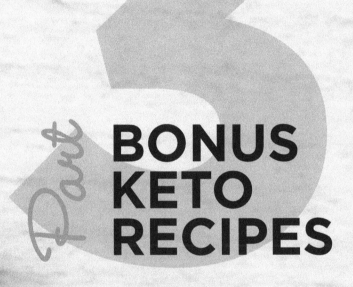

# Part 3

# BONUS KETO RECIPES

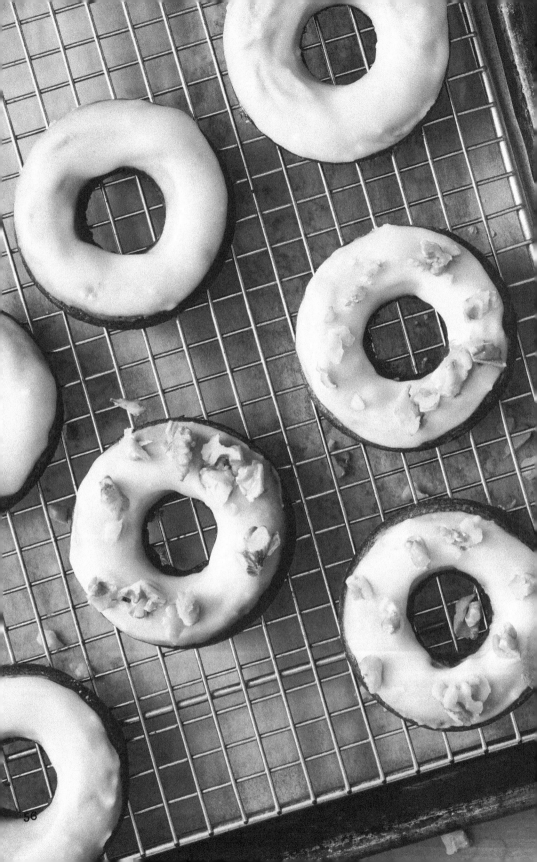

# Six
# BREAKFAST

Cinnamon-Nut Cottage Cheese 58

Cheesy Scrambled Eggs 59

French Toast Egg Muffins 60

Egg & Cheese Biscuit Casserole 62

Savory Sausage Balls 64

Chaffles 65

Biscuits with Gravy 66

Chocolate Cake Donuts 68

Chocolate Cake Donuts
**68**

# Cinnamon-Nut Cottage Cheese

**1 SERVING**

**PREP TIME:** 5 minutes

Whether you're a cottage cheese lover or not, you owe it to yourself to try this. It's literally my favorite breakfast and snack, and it's so easy to prepare. There are many variations, and it can be warmed just a bit in the microwave, although I prefer it cold. This recipe originated from my yearning for oatmeal, which is totally not keto. That craving has been tamed—crisis averted!

½ cup
**cottage cheese**

1 **stevia packet** or
a few squirts liquid
**stevia** or substitute

2 teaspoons to
1 tablespoon
**cinnamon**

¼ cup
**chopped pecans**

1. In a bowl, combine the cottage cheese and stevia, mixing well.

2. Add the cinnamon and mix just to incorporate. Add more cinnamon or stevia to taste.

3. Sprinkle the pecans on top and enjoy!

**TIP:** If you'd like to warm it up, put it in the microwave for about 20 seconds, being careful not to overcook it. You can also add berries, other nuts, or sugar-free chocolate chips. Just be sure to add the additional carbs to your total.

___

**Per Serving** Calories: 324; Total fat: 27g;

Carbohydrates: 10g; Fiber: 4g; Protein: 15g; Net carbs: 6g

# Cheesy Scrambled Eggs

**1 SERVING**

**PREP TIME:** 5 minutes / Cook time: 8 minutes

I've been a scrambled egg lover since I was a kid, but this cheesy version with savory sausage and creamy avocado takes it up a notch and is a favorite day-starter at our house. Lovies's daughter Kristina asks for them every time she comes home from college. With so many different versions available, you could eat them every day and never get bored.

1 tablespoon butter

1 tablespoon cream cheese

1 ounce cooked breakfast sausage

2 large eggs

½ teaspoon pepper

½ teaspoon garlic salt

¼ cup grated Cheddar cheese

½ avocado, sliced

1. In a small skillet over medium heat, melt the butter, then add the cream cheese. Use a spatula to mash the cream cheese and mix it well with the butter.

2. Add the breakfast sausage and mix well.

3. Add the eggs and scramble until cooked. Season with the pepper and garlic salt.

4. Top with the Cheddar cheese and avocado slices and enjoy.

**TIP:** Add any protein you'd like—ham, oven-roasted turkey, bacon, and so much more. Any cheese is delicious, and you can top it with salsa, hot sauce, or sour cream. Just be sure to add the additional carbs to your total.

**Per Serving** Calories: 614; Total fat: 54g; Carbohydrates: 8g; Fiber: 5g; Protein: 27g; Net carbs: 3g

# French Toast Egg Muffins

**12 MUFFINS**

**PREP TIME:** 10 minutes / Cook time: 20 to 25 minutes

Egg loaf, a simple but delicious loaf made with just a few ingredients, hit the keto scene a while back and quickly became a huge hit. Everyone has their own way of making it, but my favorite is as a muffin. You can also pour the whole concoction into a casserole dish and cook it up as well. It's an interesting texture—not really bread-like but not eggy either. Kind of spongy, like French toast when it's wet and gooey. Most importantly, it's a family favorite.

Nonstick cooking spray (optional)

8 large eggs

1 (8-ounce) brick cream cheese

2 tablespoons sugar-free maple syrup, plus 12 tablespoons for topping

1 tablespoon butter

1 teaspoon vanilla extract

1 teaspoon baking soda

½ teaspoon cinnamon

1. Preheat the oven to 350°F. Prepare a 12-cup muffin pan with nonstick cooking spray or cupcake liners.

2. In a blender, combine the eggs, cream cheese, 2 tablespoons of syrup, butter, vanilla, baking soda, and cinnamon and pulse until well blended.

3. Divide the mixture evenly between the prepared muffin cups. Fill the cups all the way to the top.

4. Bake for 20 to 25 minutes.

5. Allow the muffins to cool on the counter for a few minutes. Just before serving, drizzle 1 tablespoon of syrup on top of each muffin.

**TIP:** I love these hot, right out of the oven, but also on the go or right out of the refrigerator. You could also sprinkle some sugar-free confectioners' sugar on top. Alternatively, add some berries, different nuts, sugar-free chocolate chips, or unsweetened cocoa powder. Just be sure to add the additional carbs to your total.

---

**Per Serving (1 muffin)** Calories 122; Total fat: 11g; Carbohydrates: 1g; Fiber: 0g; Protein: 5g; Net carbs: 1g

---

**Per Serving (1 tablespoon sugar-free syrup)** Calories 32; Total fat: 0g; Carbohydrates: 15g; Fiber: 14g; Protein: 0g; Net carbs: 1g

# Egg & Cheese Biscuit Casserole

**9 SERVINGS**

**PREP TIME:** 15 minutes / Cook time: 20 minutes

Every Christmas, my mother used to make a casserole first thing in the morning. Layered white bread on the bottom and an egg mixture on top made for absolutely delicious memories. A couple of years ago, I figured out a way to make this nostalgic dish keto friendly, and now we eat it all the time instead of waiting for Christmas Day.

4 tablespoons (½ stick) butter, at room temperature, plus more for greasing the pan

½ cup coconut flour

2 teaspoons baking powder

¼ teaspoon salt

7 large eggs, divided

¼ cup sour cream

2 tablespoons heavy cream

1 teaspoon salt

1 teaspoon freshly ground black pepper

1 cup grated Cheddar cheese

1. Preheat the oven to 400°F. Grease a 9-by-9-inch casserole dish and set aside.

2. In a small bowl, whisk together the coconut flour, baking powder, and salt.

3. In a medium bowl, whisk together 3 eggs, the sour cream, and 4 tablespoons of butter.

4. Pour the dry mixture into the egg mixture, and mix well until just a few lumps remain.

5. Transfer the dough mixture to the casserole dish and mash to spread evenly across the bottom.

6. In a small bowl, whisk together the remaining 4 eggs and the heavy cream, salt, and pepper, and pour over the dough mixture.

7. Bake for 15 minutes. Pull the casserole out and sprinkle the Cheddar cheese across the top. Return to the oven for another 3 to 5 minutes or until the cheese is melted.

8. Allow to rest for 5 to 10 minutes before serving.

**TIP:** The variation options are endless, but one that we really love is adding a can of diced tomatoes and green chilies to the egg mixture. You can also add cooked breakfast sausage, ham, or bacon bits, and top with sour cream or salsa. Just be sure to add the additional carbs to your total.

---

**Per Serving (⅙ of casserole)** Calories 280; Total fat: 22g; Carbohydrates: 9g; Fiber: 5g; Protein: 14g; Net carbs: 4g

# Savory Sausage Balls

**PREP TIME:** 10 minutes / Cook time: 25 minutes

I used to make sausage balls for Christmas morning and other special occasions, but now they're a staple at our house. These savory and cheesy meatballs go perfectly as a breakfast side or as a snack right out of the refrigerator. Hot or cold, they're awesome either way.

1 pound
breakfast sausage

1 cup coconut flour

1½ cups shredded
mozzarella cheese
(or any other
white cheese)

1 (5.2-ounce)
package Boursin
cheese, Garlic &
Fine Herbs or any
other flavor

2 large eggs

2 tablespoons
butter, at room
temperature

2 teaspoons
baking powder

1 teaspoon
garlic salt

1. Preheat the oven to 350°F. Line a baking sheet with parchment paper.

2. In a large bowl, combine all the ingredients and mix well with your hands or a spatula.

3. Using a cookie scoop, drop a scoopful into your hand, roll into a ball, and place on the prepared baking sheet. Repeat with the remaining mixture.

4. Bake for about 25 minutes or until golden brown. Turn the baking sheet 180 degrees about halfway through the cook time and wiggle each ball so they don't stick.

5. Store the cooled meatballs in a resealable container in the refrigerator.

**TIP:** Don't have Boursin cheese? Substitute 5 ounces of cream cheese or half a can (5 ounces) of diced tomatoes and green chilies. You can also add any grated cheese you like. Just be sure to add the additional carbs to your total.

---

**Per Serving (2 sausage balls)** Calories: 254; Total fat: 19g;

Carbohydrates: 9g; Fiber: 6g; Protein: 12g; Net carbs: 3g

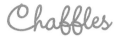
# Chaffles

**1 SERVING**

**PREP TIME:** 5 minutes / Cook time: 10 to 15 minutes

It wouldn't be a keto cookbook without the most popular new keto item of all—the chaffle! This cheese waffle can be sweet or savory, and it's a wonderful replacement for bread in sandwiches or even just garnished with a smear of cream cheese and bagel seasoning. This recipe is the basic version using the Dash Mini Waffle Maker. A larger, standard waffle iron may only make one chaffle with this recipe, or you can fill half of the waffle maker.

Nonstick cooking spray, butter, or oil for greasing the waffle maker

1 large egg

⅓ cup grated Cheddar cheese, divided

1. Grease and preheat a waffle maker.

2. In a small bowl, whisk together the egg and a third of the cheese.

3. Sprinkle some grated cheese right onto the waffle maker and add half the egg and cheese mixture. Sprinkle a little more cheese on the mixture and close the lid on the waffle maker.

4. Let the waffle cook for 4 to 5 minutes. If it's not as crispy as you'd like, flip and cook for 1 to 2 minutes more. Repeat the process with the remaining egg mixture and cheese.

**TIP:** There are so many variations for chaffles, from using different cheeses to adding blueberries or pumpkin purée. Whatever you do with your chaffle, be sure to add the additional carbs to your total. If you don't have a waffle maker, heat a little butter or oil in a skillet over medium heat and cook on each side for 4 to 5 minutes.

**Per Serving** Calories: 222; Total fat: 17g; Carbohydrates: 1g; Fiber: 0g; Protein: 16g; Net carbs: 1g

# Biscuits with Gravy

## 12 BISCUITS WITH GRAVY

**PREP TIME:** 15 minutes / Cook time: 15 minutes

Is there any better comfort food than biscuits and gravy? It took me a while to perfect this seemingly off-limits recipe, but I finally got it. You don't need to make the gravy if you're short on time and energy, but this meaty and creamy gravy adds a special touch.

### FOR THE BISCUITS

½ cup coconut flour

2 teaspoons baking powder

¼ teaspoon salt

3 large eggs

¼ cup sour cream

4 tablespoons (½ stick) butter, at room temperature

### FOR THE GRAVY

1 pound breakfast sausage

4 ounces cream cheese

1 cup heavy (whipping) cream

1 teaspoon freshly ground black pepper

### TO MAKE THE BISCUITS

1. Preheat the oven to 350°F. Line a baking sheet with parchment paper and set aside.

2. In a small bowl, whisk together the coconut flour, baking powder, and salt.

3. In a medium bowl, whisk together the eggs, sour cream, and butter.

4. Pour the dry mixture into the egg mixture and stir until well combined but still lumpy.

5. Scoop the biscuit mixture into 12 even mounds on the prepared baking sheet. Bake for 10 to 14 minutes or until golden brown.

### TO MAKE THE GRAVY

1. Meanwhile, in a skillet over medium heat, brown the breakfast sausage, then drain.

2. Add the cream cheese to the skillet and mix well.

**3.** Reduce the heat to low, add the heavy cream and pepper, and stir frequently for 10 to 15 minutes, until the gravy reaches the thickness you desire. If it gets too thick, add a little water.

**TO SERVE**

**1.** Cut a biscuit in half and spoon a tablespoon of gravy on each half.

**TIP:** These biscuits make a great snack or side to a meal. You can also add grated cheese or seasonings to create a multitude of different flavors. The biscuits taste great plain or slathered with butter or sugar-free jam. Just be sure to adjust the carb count accordingly.

---

**Per Serving (1 biscuit with 2 tablespoons gravy)** Calories: 301; Total fat: 27g; Carbohydrates: 5g; Fiber: 2g; Protein: 9g; Net carbs: 3g

---

**Per Serving (1 biscuit)** Calories: 87; Total fat: 7g; Carbohydrates: 4g; Fiber: 2g; Protein: 2g; Net carbs: 2g

---

**Per Serving (2 tablespoons gravy)** Calories: 214; Total fat: 20g; Carbohydrates: 1g; Fiber: 0g; Protein: 7g; Net carbs: 1g

# Chocolate Cake Donuts

**12 DONUTS**

**PREP TIME:** 15 minutes / Cook time: 20 minutes

Everyone loves donuts, so this recipe is sure to make any day start out a little bit better. You can even make them the night before. Chocolate is my favorite variety, so let's start there—see the tip for other flavor variation ideas. It's not mandatory, but if you have a donut pan, awesome—now is the time to use it!

Nonstick cooking spray (optional)

½ cup Lakanto Monkfruit with Erythritol (Golden) or sugar-free granulated sugar substitute (see tip)

¼ cup coconut flour

¼ cup unsweetened cocoa powder

½ teaspoon salt

¼ teaspoon baking powder

4 large eggs

8 tablespoons (1 stick) butter, at room temperature

¼ cup buttermilk

1. Preheat the oven to 350°F. Prepare a donut pan or muffin pan with nonstick cooking spray or line a baking sheet with parchment paper and set aside.

2. In a small bowl, mix together the sugar substitute, coconut flour, cocoa powder, salt, and baking powder.

3. In a medium bowl, whisk together the eggs, butter, and buttermilk.

4. Add the dry mixture to the egg mixture and mix until incorporated.

5. Scoop the batter into 12 portions in the donut or muffin pan, or fill a piping bag or a gallon-size resealable bag with a corner cut off and pipe circles onto the prepared baking sheet.

6. Bake for 15 to 20 minutes, watching closely and turning the pan halfway through the cooking time.

**TIP:** I call for Lakanto Monkfruit with Erythritol (Golden) as a sweetener, but you can use whatever sugar replacement you like; just try to use one that is a 1:1 replacement for sugar. I like these donuts plain, but you could also add a glaze by mixing a little sugar-free confectioners' sugar with a little water or sugar-free almond milk. Just play with it until you get the right consistency, starting with ¼ cup of sugar and adding the liquid slowly. Drizzle it over the donuts. You can also add nuts, sugar-free chocolate chips, unsweetened pumpkin instead of cocoa powder, blueberries, and so much more. Use your imagination; just be sure to add the additional carbs to your total.

---

**Per Serving (1 donut)** Calories: 114; Total fat: 10g; Carbohydrates: 3g; Fiber: 2g; Protein: 3g; Sugar alcohols: 8g; Net carbs: 1g

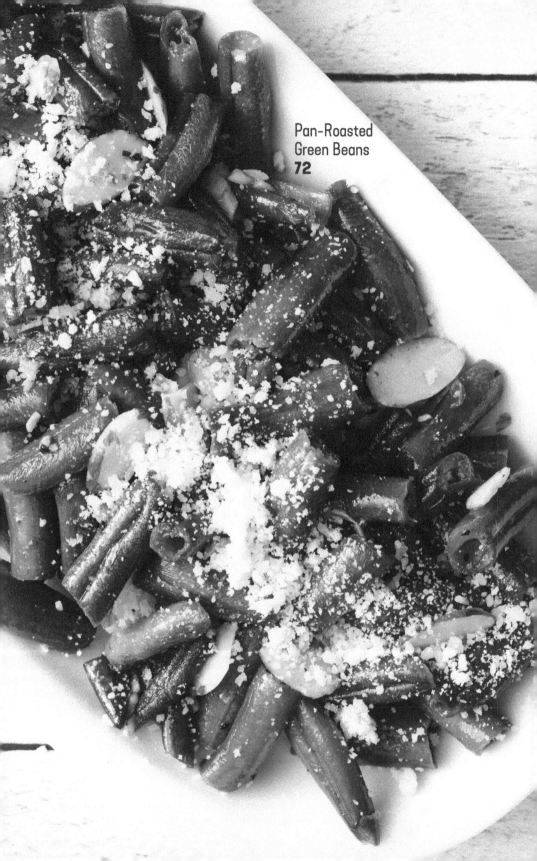

Pan-Roasted
Green Beans
**72**

# Seven
# VEGETABLES AND SIDES

# Pan-Roasted Green Beans

**4 SERVINGS**

**PREP TIME:** 5 minutes / Cook time: 15 minutes

It takes just a few ingredients to elevate green beans to star status; in this case, sliced almonds, Parmesan, garlic salt, and pepper do the trick. This dish is such a family favorite and so easy to make. I always use frozen green beans and keep three or four packages in the freezer at all times. They're so handy and can taste as good as fresh—just rinse them and pat them dry so they cook up crisp.

3 tablespoons extra-virgin olive oil

1 (12-ounce) bag frozen green beans, rinsed and patted dry

1 teaspoon garlic salt

1 teaspoon freshly ground black pepper

¼ cup sliced almonds

¼ cup grated Parmesan cheese

1. In a skillet over medium heat, heat the oil.

2. Add the green beans, garlic salt, and pepper to the skillet and cook, stirring frequently and tossing to coat, for 10 to 12 minutes.

3. Increase the heat to high and keep moving the beans around until they begin to brown.

4. Sprinkle in the almonds and stir to combine.

5. Remove from the heat, sprinkle the Parmesan cheese on top, and serve.

**TIP:** Be sure to dry the beans before putting them in the skillet so there's no additional moisture. To make this a full meal, add some chicken, sausage, or hamburger meat. Just be sure to add the additional carbs to your total.

**Per Serving (¼ recipe)** Calories: 193; Total fat: 16g; Carbohydrates: 8g; Fiber: 3g; Protein: 6g; Net carbs: 5g

# Garlic Butter Broccoli

**4 SERVINGS**

**PREP TIME:** 5 minutes / Cook time: 10 minutes

This is such a crazy easy recipe, but I had to include it because it's a big favorite and we enjoy it often. It's ready in minutes and goes with anything.

1 (12.6-ounce) microwavable bag frozen broccoli florets

3 tablespoons butter, at room temperature

1 tablespoon cream cheese, at room temperature

2 teaspoons garlic salt

1 teaspoon freshly ground black pepper

1. Microwave the broccoli according to the package instructions.

2. Remove the bag from the microwave and tear open a small corner of the bag to drain the broccoli.

3. In a small bowl, mash together the butter, cream cheese, garlic salt, and pepper, and add the mixture to the bag of broccoli.

4. Roll the top of the broccoli bag shut, and shake until the broccoli is fully coated, about a minute.

5. Pour the contents into a bowl and enjoy.

**TIP:** Usually we'll eat this as just a side, but sometimes we add hamburger meat, chicken, or sausage to turn it into a quick meal. If you do, just be sure to add the additional carbs to your total.

---

**Per Serving (¼ bag)** Calories: 111; Total fat: 10g; Carbohydrates: 4g; Fiber: 3g; Protein: 3g; Net carbs: 1g

# Oven-Roasted Brussels Sprouts & Parmesan

**4 SERVINGS**

**PREP TIME:** 10 minutes / Cook time: 40 minutes

There was a time you couldn't pay me enough money to eat a Brussels sprout, but then I learned they are amazing roasted in the oven—tender inside, crispy outside, and with a caramelized sweetness that can't be duplicated by any other cooking method. This is such a crowd pleaser and so easy to make. Join the fan club!

1 pound Brussels sprouts, trimmed and halved

¼ cup extra-virgin olive oil or ghee

1 teaspoon garlic salt

1 teaspoon freshly ground black pepper

¼ cup grated Parmesan cheese

1. Preheat the oven to 400°F. Line a baking sheet with parchment paper and set aside.

2. Place the Brussels sprouts in a gallon-size resealable bag along with the olive oil, garlic salt, and pepper.

3. Work the bag gently to completely coat each Brussels sprout.

4. Empty the Brussels sprouts onto the prepared baking sheet and spread them out in a single layer.

5. Roast for approximately 40 minutes or until golden brown. Shake the pan occasionally to roast them evenly. Watch carefully, because some of the leaves that have fallen off will brown very quickly. Remove those from the oven before they burn.

6. Remove the baking sheet from the oven and sprinkle the Brussels sprouts with the Parmesan cheese.

**TIP:** I like to buy Brussels sprouts fresh from the vegetable section, but frozen is fine, too. Just be sure to thaw them and pat them dry. These are so good by themselves when roasted that they need very few additions, but adding bacon bits on top is delicious. My favorite thing to do is put a serving in a bowl and then lay a fried egg on top and mix it all up. There usually aren't any leftovers, but if so, they're even better the next day. Just be sure to add the additional carbs to your total.

---

**Per Serving (4 ounces or ¼ pan)** Calories: 203; Total fat: 15g; Carbohydrates: 11g; Fiber: 5g; Protein: 6g; Net carbs: 6g

# Zucchini Au Gratin

**PREP TIME:** 15 minutes / Cook time: 40 minutes

This is one of my favorite recipes because it's easy, cheesy, tasty, and quickly thrown together. Bacon bits make a great topping on this dish, as well as crushed pork rinds for a little extra crunch. Just be sure to add the additional carbs to your total.

2 tablespoons butter, at room temperature, plus more for greasing the pan

6 medium (about 8 inches long by 2 inches in diameter) zucchini, thinly sliced

½ cup heavy cream

2 ounces cream cheese, at room temperature

1 teaspoon garlic salt

1 teaspoon onion powder

1 teaspoon freshly ground black pepper

2 cups grated white Cheddar cheese

1. Preheat the oven to 375°F. Lightly grease an 8-by-8-inch baking dish and set aside.

2. Divide the zucchini slices into 3 stacks and set aside.

3. Mix the heavy cream, cream cheese, 2 tablespoons of butter, garlic salt, onion powder, and pepper to make a thin paste. If it's too thick, microwave for just a few seconds or add a little more heavy cream.

4. Layer a third of the zucchini slices on the bottom of the baking the dish.

5. With a spatula or the back of a spoon, drizzle a third of the cream mixture over the zucchini.

6. Scatter a third of the white Cheddar over the mixture and layer another third of the zucchini on top of the cheese.

7. Repeat with the cream mixture and Cheddar cheese on the next layer, and
then once again with the zucchini, cream, and ending with the remaining
Cheddar cheese.

8. Bake for 40 minutes, until golden brown.

**TIP:** This dish stores easily in the refrigerator and tastes even better the next day.

**Per Serving (⅙ casserole)** Calories: 316; Total fat: 27g; Carbohydrates: 8g; Fiber: 2g; Protein: 13g; Net carbs: 6g

# Mac & Cheese

**PREP TIME:** 15 minutes / Cook time: 20 minutes

We all grew up loving macaroni and cheese, but some of us have found this delicious duo is way too high in carbs and calories. This keto-friendly, cheesy version will leave you satisfied and guilt-free all at the same time. Cauliflower is chameleon-like in its ability to fool the palate by taking on the texture and flavor of the goodies it's cooked with. Enter keto-friendly Mac & Cheese. Enjoy!

1 pound cauliflower, chopped into bite-size pieces

¼ cup heavy cream, plus more if needed

2 ounces cubed cream cheese, at room temperature

1 teaspoon garlic salt

1 teaspoon freshly ground black pepper

1 cup grated Parmesan cheese

1 cup grated white Cheddar cheese

1 cup grated sharp Cheddar cheese

¾ cup crushed pork rinds

1. Place the cauliflower in a pot of water on the stove over high heat. Bring to a boil.

2. Boil for 5 to 10 minutes or until fork-tender. Drain, reduce the heat to low, and return the cauliflower to the stove.

3. Add the heavy cream, cream cheese, garlic salt, and pepper, and mix.

4. Slowly add the Parmesan, white Cheddar, and sharp Cheddar, stirring as you go. If the mixture is too thick, add a little extra heavy cream.

5. Once all the cheese is mixed in and melted, pour the mixture into a casserole dish.

6. Just before serving, sprinkle the pork rinds on top.

**TIP:** This dish is also wonderful topped with bacon bits instead of crushed pork rinds, and it works well with all kinds of different cheeses. We've also added a drained can of diced tomatoes and green chilies, and it was great, as well. If you want additional crunch on top, add some more crushed pork rinds. Just be sure to add the additional carbs to your total.

---

**Per Serving (⅙ casserole)** Calories: 346; Total fat: 26g; Carbohydrates: 6g; Fiber: 2g; Protein: 22g; Net carbs: 4g

# Jalapeño Cream Cheese Poppers

**6 SERVINGS**

**PREP TIME:** 15 minutes / Cook time: 20 to 30 minutes

We usually make a batch of 35 jalapeños, and it's a family affair, assembly-line-style. Everyone on the team pitches in because they know these jalapeños are delicious, hot or cold. I'm going to introduce you to this recipe with six jalapeños cut in half to make six servings, with directions for both the grill and the oven. Once you make these and taste their greatness, you'll want to double or triple up for future batches.

**6 (3- to 4-inch) jalapeños, halved and seeded**

**4 ounces cream cheese**

**12 slices uncooked bacon**

1. If using the oven, preheat to 375°F and line a baking sheet with parchment paper.

2. If using the grill, set it on low and make an aluminum foil boat or use a grill mat.

3. Using a small kitchen knife or butter knife, fill each of the jalapeño halves with cream cheese.

4. Starting at the stem end of a jalapeño, lay a slice of bacon lengthwise across the cream cheese down toward the pointed end, and then wrap the bacon around the outside of the jalapeño all the way back to the stem so the entire jalapeño is wrapped in bacon and the cream cheese won't bubble out. Repeat with the remaining jalapeños.

5. To cook in the oven, place the jalapeños cream cheese–side up on the parchment paper, and bake for 20 to 30 minutes, until the bacon is crispy.

6. To cook on the grill, place the jalapeños cream cheese–side down on the foil boat or grill mat. Grill for 10 minutes, flip them over, and cook for an additional 10 minutes.

TIP: There is nothing else we do with these poppers except plate them and eat them like candy! Any leftovers that happen to sneak by are stored in the refrigerator and just as good cold. One bit of prep advice: The cream cheese and bacon are both easier to work with when they're a little closer to room temperature.

---

Per Serving (2 jalapeño halves) Calories: 155; Total fat: 13g; Carbohydrates: 2g; Fiber: 0g; Protein: 7g; Net carbs: 2g

# Bacony Green Beans

**3½ SERVINGS**

**PREP TIME:** 5 minutes / Cook time: 40 minutes

My mother made green beans when I was a kid, but they never included bacon and certainly not bacon grease! Well, these do, and they're a staple at our house as a side for just about any meal we sit down to. They're on permanent rotation in the refrigerator. And while this recipe calls for canned green beans, use any kind you wish—they're good any way you make them!

¼ **pound uncooked bacon, cut into 1-inch pieces**

1 teaspoon **seasoned salt**

1 teaspoon **freshly ground black pepper**

1 teaspoon **garlic powder**

1 (14.5-ounce) **can green beans, undrained**

¼ **medium red onion, chopped**

1. In a medium skillet over medium heat, cook the bacon.

2. Once the bacon is cooked, add the seasoned salt, pepper, and garlic powder, and stir.

3. Add the green beans and their juices, then the onion, mixing to combine.

4. Reduce the heat to low and simmer for 30 minutes, stirring occasionally.

**TIP:** We often add cooked breakfast sausage to this dish along with the bacon. It's such a great combination. If you do, just be sure to add the additional carbs to your total.

---

**Per Serving (½ cup)** Calories: 150; Total fat: 13g; Carbohydrates: 5g; Fiber: 2g; Protein: 4g; Net carbs: 3g

# Bacon Onion Rings

4 SERVINGS

**PREP TIME:** 15 minutes / Cook time: 40 minutes

These Bacon Onion Rings are the perfect side for dinner or lunch, great as a snack on the go, and especially popular to serve or take to a party. One onion will make about 12 onion rings, but they're all different—just know that a quarter of the onion rings equals one serving.

**1 large yellow onion**

**1 pound bacon**

1. Preheat the oven to 400°F. Line a baking sheet with parchment paper and set aside.

2. Peel and slice the onion into ½-inch rings, and separate the rings.

3. Starting at one side of an onion ring, wrap a slice of bacon around the onion, in and out, all the way around until you reach the beginning. The entire ring should be covered.

4. Place the onion ring on the baking sheet and repeat with the remaining onion rings.

5. Bake for 35 to 40 minutes or until crispy, flipping the onions halfway through the cooking time.

**TIP:** The bacon is easier to work with when it's a little softer, not straight out of the refrigerator, so take it out about 15 minutes prior to wrapping. Cooked onion rings are great dipped in ranch dressing or with additional seasonings sprinkled on top. Just be sure to add the additional carbs to your total.

---

**Per Serving (about 3 onion rings)** Calories: 188; Total fat: 13g; Carbohydrates: 4g; Fiber: 1g; Protein: 12g; Net carbs: 3g

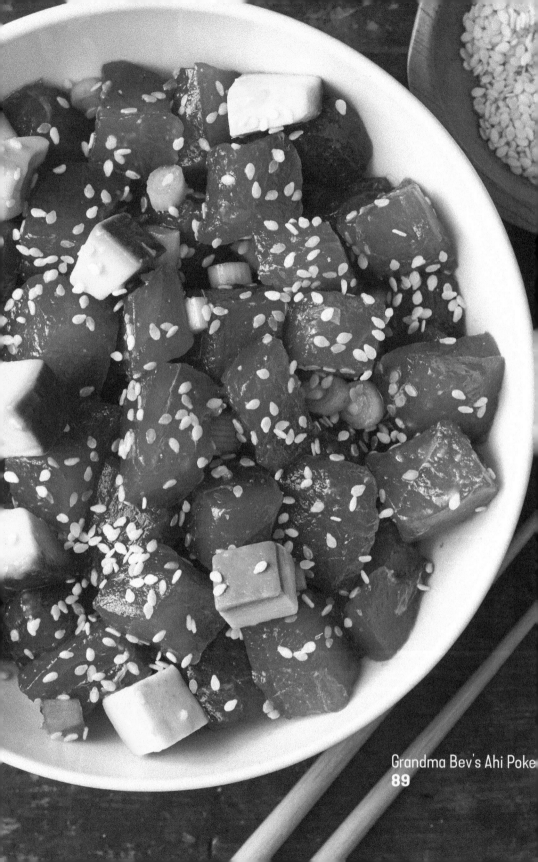

Grandma Bev's Ahi Poke

# *Eight*
# SEAFOOD ENTRÉES

# Sheet-Pan Shrimp

**4 SERVINGS**

**PREP TIME:** 15 minutes / Cook time: 10 minutes

Shrimp always make such a pretty meal and can be added to just about anything. I love the ease of this sheet-pan recipe, and it's absolutely delicious, as well. Spread some sliced zucchini or summer squash around the outside of the pan to make this a complete meal.

**8 tablespoons (1 stick) butter, melted**

**4 ounces cream cheese, at room temperature**

**1 teaspoon garlic salt**

**1 pound shrimp, any size, peeled, deveined, tails off, patted dry**

**Juice of 1 lemon**

**2 scallions, thinly sliced**

1. Preheat the oven to 400°F. Line a rimmed baking sheet with parchment paper and set aside.

2. In a medium bowl, mix together the melted butter, cream cheese, and garlic salt until well combined.

3. Drop the shrimp into the butter mixture and fold gently to coat all the shrimp.

4. Pour the shrimp mixture onto the prepared baking sheet and spread out the shrimp so none overlap.

5. Bake for 8 to 10 minutes.

6. Squeeze the lemon juice across the top of the shrimp, garnish with the scallions, and serve immediately.

**TIP:** I also love this dish with a can of diced tomatoes and green chilies (drained) poured across the top of the shrimp or with a generous sprinkle of Parmesan cheese. Another option is to cut an avocado in half and fill one side with the shrimp. Just be sure to add the additional carbs to your total.

**Per Serving (¼ recipe)** Calories: 420; Total fat: 35g; Carbohydrates: 3g; Fiber: 0g; Protein: 25g; Net carbs: 3g

# Bacon-Wrapped Shrimp

**4 SERVINGS**

**PREP TIME:** 10 minutes / Cook time: 15 minutes

Of course, bacon-wrapped anything is delicious, but bacon-wrapped shrimp are especially so. They make for a savory meal, snack, or party appetizer that never disappoints. These are also about the easiest thing in the world to make. Pair this dish with a nice salad or zucchini noodles for a complete meal.

**1 pound shrimp, peeled, deveined, tails still attached**

**20 slices bacon**

1. Preheat the oven to 400°F. Line a baking sheet with parchment paper.

2. Wrap each shrimp with a slice of bacon, secure with a toothpick, and place on the prepared baking sheet.

3. Bake about 15 minutes or until the bacon looks crispy.

**TIP:** I like to flip the shrimp about halfway through the baking time to get both sides crispy. A fun addition is to drizzle sugar-free maple syrup across them once you take them out of the oven. The syrup really takes the flavor and presentation up a notch for parties! Just be sure to add the additional carbs to your total.

---

**Per Serving (about 5 shrimp)** Calories: 335; Total fat: 19g; Carbohydrates: 2g; Fiber: 0g; Protein: 38g; Net carbs: 2g

# Grandma Kitty's Tuna Salad

**4 SERVINGS**

**PREP TIME:** 10 minutes

Tuna salad has been a favorite of mine for as long as I can remember, and my mama made the best. Whenever she came to visit, she always brought my son Zack one of his favorite food dishes to put in the refrigerator, and this was definitely his favorite. She never came empty-handed. Directions for hard-boiling eggs are included in the Buttery Boiled Eggs recipe on page 44 (steps 1 to 4).

3 (6-ounce) cans white albacore tuna in water, well drained

3 large hard-boiled eggs

1 small dill pickle

1 teaspoon seasoned salt

1 teaspoon garlic salt

1 teaspoon freshly ground black pepper

¼ cup mayonnaise

¼ cup sour cream

1. Place the well-drained tuna into a medium bowl and use a fork to break up the chunks.

2. Chop the hard-boiled eggs and pickle, and add them to the tuna.

3. Add the seasoned salt, garlic salt, and pepper, and mix well.

4. Add the mayonnaise and sour cream, and mix well.

**TIP:** Mom added black olives to her version, which was also great. If you'd like to try it, just chop up and add 6 to 8 large black olives. My favorite way to eat this tuna salad is on a bed of lettuce or stuffed in half of an avocado with a little ranch dressing drizzled on top. Feel free to do the same—just be sure to add the additional carbs to your total.

**Per Serving (¼ recipe)** Calories: 276; Total fat: 12g; Carbohydrates: 4g; Fiber: 0g; Protein: 35g; Net carbs: 4g

# Grandma Bev's Ahi Poke

**6 SERVINGS**

**PREP TIME:** 10 minutes

If you enjoy sushi and sashimi, make your own at home in a flash. Even though this native Hawaiian dish is trending right now, my dad's sweet wife Bev (Grandma Bev to the grandkids) introduced this ahi poke recipe to me 15 years ago or more. She loves to send some home with me after I visit her and my dad, to share with Lovies and the kids, but it rarely ever makes it home. Just too good to share!

**3 scallions, diced**

**½ cup soy sauce**

**2 teaspoons sesame oil**

**1 tablespoon sesame seeds**

**¼ teaspoon ground ginger**

**1 teaspoon garlic powder**

**1 teaspoon salt**

**2 pounds fresh ahi tuna, cut into ½-inch cubes**

1. In a medium bowl, mix the scallions, soy sauce, sesame oil, sesame seeds, ginger, garlic powder, and salt.

2. Combine the soy sauce mixture with the tuna, and toss well. Serve immediately.

3. If not serving immediately, store the tuna and the soy sauce mixture separately in the refrigerator until ready to serve.

**TIP:** This dish is perfect just the way it is as an appetizer, light meal, or party tray, but if you want to kick it up a notch, you could add crushed red pepper flakes or chili sauce. I also like to add cut-up chunks of avocado. Just be sure to add the additional carbs to your total.

**Per Serving (⅙ recipe)** Calories: 241; Total fat: 9g; Carbohydrates: 2g; Fiber: 1g; Protein: 38g; Net carbs: 1g

# Baked Tilapia & Parmesan

**PREP TIME:** 10 minutes / Cook time: 15 minutes

Tilapia and Parmesan are two ingredients that really go well together and make such a lovely light lunch or dinner. The crunchy addition of crushed pork rinds on top makes it out-of-this-world delicious. Enjoy this as a meal alongside some spaghetti squash or green beans.

**4 tablespoons (½ stick) butter, melted**

**2 teaspoons garlic salt**

**1 teaspoon freshly ground black pepper**

**4 (4-ounce) tilapia fillets, patted dry**

**4 ounces grated Parmesan cheese**

**4 ounces crushed pork rinds**

1. Preheat the oven to 400°F. Line a baking sheet with parchment paper and set aside.

2. In a small bowl, mix the melted butter, garlic salt, and pepper. Place the tilapia fillets on the prepared baking sheet, then drizzle or brush the butter mixture across each fillet.

3. Sprinkle each fillet with Parmesan cheese and crushed pork rinds.

4. Bake for about 13 minutes, and then turn the oven up to broil and broil for 2 more minutes.

**TIP:** I don't do anything extra to this recipe, but my son loves to squeeze lemon juice across the top of his and swears it makes the dish perfect. You could also try different cheeses or add extra crushed pork rinds if you'd like it crispier. Just be sure to add the additional carbs to your total.

---

**Per Serving (1 fillet)** Calories: 372; Total fat: 24g; Carbohydrates: 1g; Fiber: 0g; Protein: 38g; Net carbs: 1g

# Crispy Fried Cod

**4 SERVINGS**

**PREP TIME:** 15 minutes / Cook time: 15 minutes

Growing up, fried fish was one of my favorite comfort foods. Even though this cod is crispy, tender, and flavorful, this version actually plays off the cafeteria version I loved as a kid, smothered in ketchup. I assure you, it's delicious!

1 cup crushed pork rinds

¼ cup grated Parmesan cheese

½ cup heavy cream

1 large egg

4 (4-ounce) cod fillets, patted dry

Extra-virgin olive oil, for frying

1 (10-ounce) can original Ro-Tel (drained)

2 tablespoons lemon juice (optional)

1. In a small bowl, combine the pork rinds and grated Parmesan.

2. In another bowl, whisk together the heavy cream and egg.

3. Dip each cod fillet completely in the egg mixture, then dip on both sides into the pork rind mixture, making sure the entire fillet is covered. Place the fillets on a plate and refrigerate while the oil heats.

4. In a heavy skillet over medium heat, heat 2 to 3 inches of oil.

5. Heat the oil to 365°F. (Dip a wooden spoon into the oil. If the oil steadily bubbles around the wooden spoon, it's ready.)

6. Working in batches if necessary, fry each fillet for about 2 minutes on each side or until the outside is golden brown.

7. Drain on a paper towel if needed, then plate and serve, topping each fillet with one-quarter of the can of Ro-Tel.

CONTINUED

# CRISPY FRIED COD CONTINUED

**TIP:** Feel free to leave out the Ro-Tel and go traditional, just squirting some lemon juice across the top. This crispy cod is also great to dip in sugar-free ketchup or sugar-free tartar sauce. Just be sure to add any additional carbs to your total.

---

**Per Serving (1 fillet)** Calories: 375; Total fat: 28g; Carbohydrates: 6g; Fiber: 0g;
Protein: 36g; Net carbs: 6g

# Pecan-Crusted Salmon

**PREP TIME:** 5 minutes / Cook time: 15 minutes

There's something about this dish that always makes me wonder why we don't make it more often. It's simple, easy, and so tasty. It makes the perfect light lunch or dinner and always seems so fancy. It's a wonderful keto meal, too, packed with nutrition and good, healthy fats.

1 tablespoon butter, melted, plus more for greasing the pan

12 ounces fresh salmon

½ cup finely chopped pecans

4 tablespoons grated Parmesan cheese

2 tablespoons cream cheese, at room temperature

1 teaspoon garlic salt

1 teaspoon freshly ground black pepper

1. Preheat the oven to 425°F. Lightly grease a 13-by-9-inch baking dish.

2. Place the salmon skin-side down in the dish.

3. In a small bowl, mix the pecans, Parmesan cheese, cream cheese, melted butter, garlic salt, and pepper, and spread evenly over the top of the salmon.

4. Bake for about 15 minutes or until the salmon flakes easily with a fork.

**TIP:** This recipe is one of those dishes that need no adjustments, and I usually just pair it with some steamed asparagus or broccoli as a meal. Just be sure to add any additional carbs to your total.

**Per Serving (3 ounces)** Calories: 303; Total fat: 24g; Carbohydrates: 3g; Fiber: 1g; Protein: 21g; Net carbs: 2g

# Salmon Cakes

**PREP TIME:** 10 minutes / Cook time: 15 minutes

My mother made salmon cakes all the time when we were kids and always used saltine crackers as the binder. They were amazing, but they didn't work with the keto diet. Now that I've replaced the crackers with almond flour and pork rinds, salmon cakes are back on the menu and better than ever.

1 (16-ounce) can pink salmon, drained and bones removed

¼ cup almond flour

¼ cup crushed pork rinds

2 scallions, diced

1 large egg

3 tablespoons mayonnaise

1 teaspoon garlic salt

1 teaspoon freshly ground black pepper

2 tablespoons extra-virgin olive oil

1. Line a plate with paper towels and set aside.

2. In a bowl, combine the salmon, almond flour, pork rinds, scallions, egg, mayonnaise, garlic salt, and pepper, and mix together well, using your hands or a spatula.

3. Form 8 small patties or 4 large patties. If the patties seem too dry, add a little more mayonnaise. If they seem too wet, add a little more almond flour or pork rinds.

4. In a skillet over medium heat, heat the oil. Cook the patties for 4 to 5 minutes on each side, until crispy. Larger patties may need to cook a little longer.

5. Transfer the patties to the lined plate to drain.

**TIP:** One of the best ways to serve these salmon cakes is with a squirt of lemon or a drizzle of Sriracha or Sarayo Sauce. You can also spice them up a bit by adding chopped jalapeños or green chiles when you make the patties. Just be sure to add any additional carbs to your total.

---

**Per Serving (2 small patties or 1 large patty)** Calories: 313; Total fat: 21g; Carbohydrates: 5g; Fiber: 0g; Protein: 26g; Net carbs: 5g

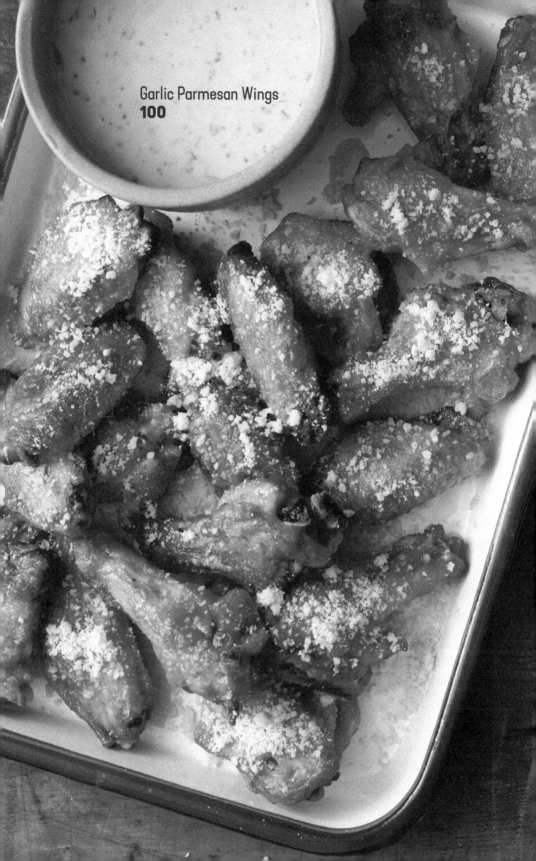

Garlic Parmesan Wings
**100**

# *Nine*
# POULTRY AND MEAT ENTRÉES

# Party Deli Pinwheels

**2 SERVINGS**

**PREP TIME:** 10 minutes, plus 5 to 10 minutes to chill

What's one of my favorite light and easy meals? Those fancy rolled-up pinwheels that they serve at parties. Here's a casual, keto-friendly version that will answer that little sandwich craving calling your name.

1 low-carb tortilla

3 tablespoons cream cheese, at room temperature

2 ounces (2 or 3 slices) oven roasted turkey

2 ounces (2 or 3 slices) fresh smoked uncured ham

2 slices provolone cheese

2 slices Cheddar cheese

1. Lay the tortilla on a plate and spread with the cream cheese.

2. Layer the meats and cheeses around the tortilla until it's covered.

3. Roll the tortilla up and refrigerate for 5 to 10 minutes or longer.

4. Cut the roll into 8 slices and serve on a plate or platter.

**TIP:** These pinwheels are great to slice and serve for parties, but you could also just eat them like a burrito. They're ideal for lunch, a light dinner, or on the go. A low-carb tortilla is the perfect launching pad for endless combinations of meats, cheeses, and toppings—try lettuce, olives, onions, avocado, roasted garlic—you name it. You could also substitute Boursin cheese, mayonnaise, or mustard for the cream cheese. Just be sure to add the additional carbs to your total.

**Per Serving (4 pinwheels)** Calories: 484; Total fat: 32g; Carbohydrates: 18g; Fiber: 9g; Protein: 31g; Net carbs: 9g

# Chicken Tenders

**4 SERVINGS**

**PREP TIME:** 10 minutes / Cook time: 25 to 30 minutes

For lunch, dinner, or a snack, chicken tenders are just the best, and that's something I think the whole family can agree on. This recipe is easy to make and yields tenders that are so crunchy and flavorful.

**2 cups crushed pork rinds**

**¼ cup grated Parmesan cheese**

**1 teaspoon garlic powder**

**1 teaspoon freshly ground black pepper**

**1 large egg**

**½ cup heavy cream**

**1 pound boneless skinless chicken tenderloins (10 to 12 tenderloins), patted dry**

1. Preheat the oven to 425°F. Line a baking sheet with parchment paper and set aside.

2. In a shallow bowl, mix the pork rinds, Parmesan cheese, garlic powder, and pepper.

3. In a separate bowl, whisk together the egg and heavy cream.

4. Dip a tenderloin entirely in the egg mixture, then lay the tenderloin in the pork rind mixture, turning to coat both sides.

5. Lay the coated tenderloin on the prepared baking sheet and repeat with the remaining tenderloins.

6. Bake for 25 to 30 minutes.

**TIP:** When you lay the tenderloins in the pork rind mixture, sprinkle some on places that don't get covered or pat it on the tenderloin to secure the mixture. These tenders taste great on their own or with ranch or blue cheese dressing. Just be sure to add the additional carbs to your total.

---

**Per Serving (3 tenderloins)** Calories: 460; Total fat: 32g; Carbohydrates: 2g; Fiber: 0g; Protein: 41g; Net carbs: 2g

# Garlic Parmesan Wings

**PREP TIME:** 5 minutes / Cook time: 1 hour

Bone-in garlic parmesan wings from Wingstop may be my most favorite food ever, and thankfully, they are so keto friendly. Here's my super easy at-home version. Go ahead and recreate the whole wing takeout experience by serving them up with celery sticks and blue cheese or ranch dressing.

**2½ pounds party chicken wing pieces (20 to 22 wings), patted dry**

**8 tablespoons (1 stick) butter, melted**

**1 tablespoon garlic salt or 1 tablespoon minced garlic**

**½ cup grated Parmesan cheese**

**1.** Preheat the oven to 375°F. Line a rimmed baking sheet with parchment paper.

**2.** Place the chicken wings on the parchment paper.

**3.** Bake for 1 hour, flipping the wings halfway through the cooking time.

**4.** Remove the chicken wings from the oven and place them in a large bowl.

**5.** Gently toss the wings in the butter and garlic salt.

**6.** Top with the grated Parmesan cheese.

**TIP:** You can give these some spice with Sriracha sauce or hot sauce. Just be sure to add the additional carbs to your total.

**Per Serving (4 chicken wings)** Calories: 469; Total fat: 40g; Carbohydrates: 1g; Fiber: 0g; Protein: 26g; Net carbs: 1g

# Bacon-Wrapped Jalapeño Chicken

**6 SERVINGS**

**PREP TIME:** 20 minutes / Cook time: 45 minutes

My partner, Lovies, started making these a few years ago, and as simple as they are, we are obsessed. He loves to cook them on his REC TEC grill, but I'm an oven girl, so this is something easy and delicious that I can do on my own indoors. Our boys, Chris and Zack, love them. We usually make a double or triple batch for the week, since they go fast!

2 tablespoons seasoned salt

2 tablespoons garlic powder

2 tablespoons freshly ground black pepper

1 pound boneless skinless chicken tenderloins (10 to 12 tenderloins), patted dry

10 to 12 slices uncooked bacon

3 jalapeños, seeded and cut lengthwise into 4 slices

1. Preheat the oven to 375°F. Line a rimmed baking sheet with parchment paper and set aside.

2. In a small bowl, mix together the seasoned salt, garlic powder, and pepper.

3. Lay a tenderloin in the seasonings, then remove it. Lay a slice of jalapeño across the tenderloin, and wrap both the chicken and the jalapeño with a slice of bacon. Place the wrapped tenderloin on the prepared baking sheet. Repeat with the remaining tenderloins.

4. Bake for 45 minutes.

**TIP:** The bacon tends to cook a little more evenly if you turn each tenderloin over about halfway through the cooking time. We store them in a resealable bag in the refrigerator, and I love to grab one as I walk out the door to eat on the go.

**Per Serving (2 tenderloins)** Calories: 303; Total fat: 22g; Carbohydrates: 2g; Fiber: 0g; Protein: 23g; Net carbs: 2g

# Sausage Egg Roll in a Bowl

**4 SERVINGS**

**PREP TIME:** 5 minutes / Cook time: 20 minutes

When you're in the mood for something different, this Asian-inspired dish tastes as savory and delicious as it sounds. It's easy to make and goes fast, too, so we usually make a double batch.

**1 pound pork breakfast sausage**

**1 (1-pound) bag shredded cabbage or coleslaw mix**

**3 tablespoons soy sauce**

**3 garlic cloves, minced**

**1 tablespoon sesame oil**

**2 scallions, thinly sliced**

1. In a skillet over medium heat, cook the breakfast sausage. Drain the grease.

2. Add the cabbage mix, soy sauce, garlic cloves, and sesame oil to the skillet with the sausage and mix well.

3. Cook for 5 to 10 minutes, until the cabbage is tender. Sprinkle with the scallions and serve warm.

**TIP:** You can add some sesame seeds for texture, and if you want some heat, Sriracha or red pepper flakes. You can also swap in any meat you choose. Just be sure to add the additional carbs to your total.

---

**Per Serving (¼ skillet)** Calories: 412; Total fat: 33g; Carbohydrates: 9g; Fiber: 3g; Protein: 20g; Net carbs: 6g

# Creole Sausage & Rice

**4 SERVINGS**

**PREP TIME:** 10 minutes / Cook time: 30 minutes

A favorite Southern comfort food is sausage and rice, which I think is even better if it's Cajun inspired. Cauliflower rice stands in nicely for regular rice. There's a lot more you could add to this dish to make a bigger meal, but if you want simple, tasty, and satisfying, this is it!

**1 teaspoon extra-virgin olive oil**

**1 pound cooked Italian sausage**

**1 (10-ounce) bag frozen cauliflower rice, thawed, rinsed, and patted dry**

**3 tablespoons chopped red onion**

**2 scallions, thinly sliced**

**1 cup chicken broth or bone broth**

**2 teaspoons Creole seasoning**

**1.** In a skillet over medium heat, heat the oil. Brown the cooked sausage for a few minutes.

**2.** Add the cauliflower rice, red onion, scallions, broth, and Creole seasoning to the skillet with the sausage and mix to incorporate all the ingredients. Cook and stir until heated through. Serve hot.

**TIP:** This dish tastes even better the next day. Feel free to toss in some chicken and shrimp, along with any other heat or spice additions you want to make. Just be sure to add the additional carbs to your total.

**Per Serving (¼ skillet)** Calories: 426; Total fat: 32g; Carbohydrates: 10g; Fiber: 2g; Protein: 24g; Net carbs: 8g

# Baked Crustless Pizza

**2 SERVINGS**

**PREP TIME:** 5 minutes / Cook time: 20 minutes

When I go to a pizza restaurant, I always order their "make your own" and choose my toppings. I also ask for no marinara sauce and no crust. It comes out different at every single restaurant but always tastes delicious. My favorite place is Luigi's, here in our hometown of Rockwall. I think their version is the best, and so this recipe is my valiant attempt to recreate it.

**8 ounces chopped Italian sausage**

**15 slices pepperoni**

**10 large black olives, sliced**

**½ cup grated mozzarella cheese**

1. Preheat the oven to 350°F.

2. In a skillet over medium heat, cook the sausage. Drain the grease and spread the sausage on the bottom of an 8-by-8-inch baking dish or pie pan.

3. Layer the pepperoni slices, black olives, and cheese over the sausage.

4. Bake, covered, for 10 to 15 minutes or until the cheese is melted and hot throughout.

**TIP:** There are so many different possible variations on this recipe; just use your imagination. You can add hamburger, chicken, or Canadian bacon, as well as onions, peppers, green olives, mushrooms, jalapeños, or anchovies. Any cheese varieties are great, as well. If you're missing the sauce, Alfredo is naturally keto friendly and amazing. My favorite is Bertolli's Garlic Alfredo. Just be sure to add the additional carbs to your total.

**Per Serving (½ skillet)** Calories: 480; Total fat: 40g; Carbohydrates: 3g; Fiber: 1g; Protein: 27g; Net carbs: 2g

# Broccoli & Beef Casserole

**4 SERVINGS**

**PREP TIME:** 15 minutes / Cook time: 30 minutes

This combo of broccoli and beef is one of my constant cravings, and this casserole version is my favorite. It's a complete meal that will keep you full, plus it always tastes so good—and even better the next day.

**1 pound ground beef**

**1 (16-ounce) bag frozen broccoli baby florets**

**1 (8-ounce) brick cream cheese**

**¼ cup ranch dressing**

**¼ cup mayonnaise**

**1 cup shredded mozzarella cheese**

**1 teaspoon Italian seasoning**

**1 tablespoon garlic salt**

**1 teaspoon freshly ground black pepper**

**¼ cup Parmesan cheese**

1. In a large skillet over medium heat, cook the ground beef, breaking up any big pieces. Drain the grease.

2. Meanwhile, microwave the broccoli according to the package directions. Drain the liquid, pat the broccoli dry, and chop the broccoli into bite-size chunks.

3. Add the broccoli, cream cheese, ranch dressing, mayonnaise, mozzarella cheese, Italian seasoning, garlic salt, and pepper to the skillet with the meat, mix together, reduce the heat to low, and cook for about 20 minutes, stirring occasionally.

4. Sprinkle the Parmesan on top and serve.

**TIP:** For a fancier presentation, transfer the casserole mixture from the skillet to a baking dish and then sprinkle on the Parmesan to serve. Another one of my favorite toppings is French's fried onions. They're not super low in carbs, but you don't need a lot. Just be sure to add the additional carbs to your total.

---

**Per Serving (¼ skillet)** Calories: 607; Total fat: 51g; Carbohydrates: 9g; Fiber: 3g; Protein: 28g; Net carbs: 6g

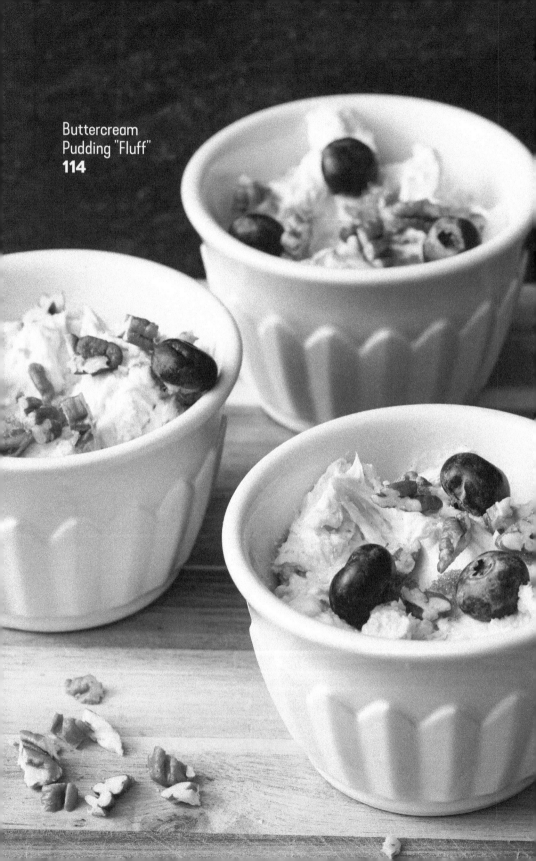

Buttercream
Pudding "Fluff"
**114**

# Ten
# SNACKS AND TREATS

# Parmesan Crisps

**6 SERVINGS**

**PREP TIME:** 5 minutes / Cook time: 5 minutes

Parmesan Crisps are the ultimate crispy keto chip! They're great by themselves or to add some crunch to salads or soups, but they really won my heart with their dipping abilities, from guacamole to peanut butter and everything in between. And they're just one ingredient!

**1 cup grated Parmesan cheese**

1. Preheat the oven to 400°F. Line a baking sheet with parchment paper.

2. With a spoon or your fingers, drop mounds of cheese onto the parchment paper and pat them down, approximately one inch apart. Alternatively, spread the cheese to cover the entire parchment paper.

3. Place the baking sheet in the oven and set the timer for 5 minutes. Watch closely, as ovens differ and the crisps brown up quickly.

4. Remove from the oven and allow to cool before removing from the pan. If the mixture was spread to cover the pan, break into pieces once cooled.

5. Store in an airtight container at room temperature for a few days or in the vegetable drawer of the refrigerator for up to a week.

**TIP:** My favorite way to eat Parmesan Crisps is with peanut butter. I grew up eating Lance brand cheese and peanut butter crackers, and that's exactly what this combo tastes like! You can also add seasonings to the cheese or even mix different cheeses together. Consider adding pepperoni or cooked breakfast sausage or chicken to the little piles of cheese and making them into little pizzas. They're also perfect for dipping into just about anything, so have fun with these crispy treats. Just be sure to add the additional carbs to your total.

---

**Per Serving (⅙ recipe)** Calories 72; Total fat: 5g; Carbohydrates: 1g; Fiber: 0g; Protein: 6g; Net carbs: 1g

# 90-Second Bread

**PREP TIME:** 5 minutes / Cook time: 90 seconds

I can't take credit for inventing 90-second bread, but I also couldn't leave it out of this book, because you will love and use it in so many ways as a replacement for bread. I do think my version is pretty good!

1 heaping tablespoon coconut flour

½ teaspoon baking powder

1 large egg

1½ tablespoons butter, melted

Pinch salt

1. In a small, 3- to 4-inch diameter, microwave-safe bowl, combine the coconut flour, baking powder, egg, butter, and salt, and mix until well combined.

2. Place the bowl in the microwave and cook on high for 90 seconds.

3. Dump the bread from the bowl and allow to cool for a couple of minutes.

4. With a serrated knife, cut the bread in half horizontally to make two halves, if desired.

**TIP:** I love sandwiches, and that's my favorite use for this recipe, but this bread is also great toasted with fried eggs on top or smeared with sugar-free jelly. Just be sure to add the additional carbs to your total.

---

**Per Serving** Calories: 204; Total fat: 17g;

Carbohydrates: 5g; Fiber: 3g; Protein: 8g; Net carbs: 2g

# Cinnamon-Glazed Pecans

**10 SERVINGS**

**PREP TIME:** 5 minutes / Cook time: 25 to 30 minutes

I love having snacks around that seem a little fancy, and these glazed pecans are perfect! They remind me so much of the delicious versions roasting at different event venues here in the South—they smell so amazing.

8 tablespoons (1 stick) butter

2½ cups pecan halves

1 teaspoon vanilla extract

2 teaspoons cinnamon

1 cup sugar-free granulated sugar

1. Line a baking sheet with parchment paper and set aside.

2. In a skillet over medium heat, melt the butter.

3. Add the pecans, vanilla, and cinnamon, and cook, stirring occasionally, for 2 minutes. Reduce the heat to low and cook, stirring occasionally, for another 10 minutes.

4. Add the sweetener and cook for another 10 to 15 minutes, until the pecans take on a glazed look.

5. Empty onto the prepared baking sheet and let cool. Once cooled, store in a resealable bag at room temperature or in the refrigerator.

**TIP:** For sweetener, I use Lakanto Monkfruit with Erythritol (Golden), but any brand you choose is fine, as long as it's a granular version that is a 1:1 replacement for sugar.

**Per Serving (¼ cup)** Calories: 289; Total fat: 29g; Carbohydrates: 4g; Fiber: 3g; Protein: 3g; Sugar alcohols: 19g; Net carbs: 1g

# Cream Cheese & Berries

**PREP TIME:** 5 minutes

Breakfast is an important part of my day, but sometimes I get tired of eggs and want something different. An easy favorite is cream cheese and berries—so tasty and refreshing and it makes a great snack.

**2 ounces cream cheese**

**2 large strawberries, cut into thin slices or chunks**

**5 blueberries**

**⅛ cup chopped pecans**

1. Place the cream cheese on a small plate or in a bowl.

2. Pour the berries and chopped pecans on top. Enjoy!

**TIP:** You can add any nuts or berries you like, or even some unsweetened coconut or sugar-free chocolate chips. Just be sure to add the additional carbs to your total.

---

**Per Serving** Calories: 330; Total fat: 31g;

Carbohydrates: 7g; Fiber: 2g; Protein: 6g; Net carbs: 5g

# Macadamia Nut Cream Cheese Log

**8 SERVINGS**

**PREP TIME:** 10 minutes, plus 30 minutes to chill

Cream cheese rolls are keto friendly and fun to create. I discovered them in Mexico. They're always on the breakfast buffet cut into slices and rolled in pecans, macadamias, sesame seeds, or other seeds or nuts.

1 (8-ounce) brick cream cheese, cold

1 cup finely chopped macadamia nuts

1. Place the cream cheese on a piece of parchment paper or wax paper.

2. Roll the paper around the cream cheese, then roll the wrapped cream cheese with the palm of your hands lengthwise on the cream cheese, using the paper to help you roll the cream cheese into an 8-inch log.

3. Open the paper and sprinkle the macadamia nuts all over the top and sides of the cream cheese until the log is entirely covered in nuts.

4. Chill in the refrigerator for 30 minutes before serving.

5. Serve on a small plate, cut into 8 even slices.

**TIP:** For variation, you could roll the cream cheese log in crushed nuts, seeds, sugar-free chopped chocolate, or any other sugar-free treat. Just be sure to add the additional carbs to your total.

**Per Serving (⅛ roll)** Calories: 285; Total fat: 29g; Carbohydrates: 4g; Fiber: 1g; Protein: 4g; Net carbs: 3g

# Buttercream Pudding "Fluff"

**10 SERVINGS**

**PREP TIME:** 10 minutes

I used to buy tubs of icing at the grocery store just to eat the icing, a spoonful at a time. When I had my specialty cake business, I had to taste-test every single bit of buttercream I made to ensure it tasted just right (perk of the job)! So when I figured out a way to hack buttercream, keto hit a whole new level of greatness. My nickname for it is "fluff," and it can be made in infinite flavors.

2½ (8-ounce) bricks cream cheese, at room temperature

8 tablespoons (1 stick) butter

1 tablespoon cinnamon

1 teaspoon vanilla extract

1 squirt liquid stevia

½ cup chopped pecans

2 tablespoons sugar-free brown sugar (see tip)

1. Using a hand mixer, whip together the cream cheese, butter, cinnamon, vanilla, and liquid stevia.

2. Gently fold in the chopped pecans and brown sugar until just incorporated.

3. Pour the mixture into a casserole or baking dish, or divide into 10 small serving bowls.

4. Store in the refrigerator until ready to serve.

**TIP:** Make sure your sugar-free brown sugar is a 1:1 replacement for real sugar. Swerve has a new brown sugar replacement that works great! You can also add a pinch of the brown sugar on top for decoration. The best part about this recipe is that it can be made so many ways! The base of the recipe is the butter and cream cheese. Whatever else you want to add to that is up to you. I enjoy it with just a squirt of stevia, but you can also add berries, nuts, sugar-free chocolate chips, and different flavorings—it's especially good with some homemade sugar-free whipped cream on top. Just be sure to add the additional carbs to your total.

---

**Per Serving (⅓ cup)** Calories: 329; Total fat: 33g; Carbohydrates: 3g; Fiber: 1g; Protein: 5g; Sugar alcohols: 4.8g; Net carbs: 2g

# Easy Peasy Peanut Butter Cookies

**PREP TIME:** 15 minutes / Cook time: 7 to 12 minutes

Peanut butter and jelly were staples for many of us growing up, and you can bet that most pantries today contain a jar or two, but how many of us have discovered real peanut butter? A few years ago, I figured out how to go to the bulk aisle of the grocery store and use their machine to make my own. All I can say is, go to the grocery store, find the bulk aisle, and make yourself some raw, real peanut butter. And then quickly make this delicious cookie recipe!

½ **cup coconut flour**

¼ **cup sugar-free sweetener (see tip)**

½ **teaspoon baking soda**

**4 tablespoons (low-carb or handmade) peanut butter**

**2 tablespoons butter, at room temperature**

**2 large eggs**

**1 teaspoon vanilla extract**

1. Preheat the oven to 350°F. Line a baking sheet with parchment paper and set aside.

2. In a bowl, combine the flour, sweetener, and baking soda, mixing to blend.

3. Add the peanut butter, butter, eggs, and vanilla, and mix well to incorporate.

4. Drop by even spoonfuls onto the prepared baking sheet to make 15 cookies.

5. Using the back of a fork, press the cookies down a little and make decorative criss-cross marks.

6. Cook for 7 to 8 minutes for soft cookies or 10 to 12 minutes for crispy cookies.

**TIP:** For sweetener, I use Lakanto Monkfruit with Erythritol (Golden), but you can use whichever brand you like. Just try to pick one that is a 1:1 replacement for real sugar. These are wonderful to make in advance and store the dough. They're easy to scoop from frozen, and then you can have them available all the time. Add sugar-free chocolate chips or chunks, macadamia nuts, or pecans, or maybe even a smear of sugar-free grape jelly on top. Just be sure to add any additional carbs to your total.

---

**Per Serving (1 cookie)** Calories: 70; Total fat: 5g; Carbohydrates: 3.2g; Fiber: 1.8g; Protein: 3g; Net carbs: 1.4g; Erythritol Carbs: 3g

# Snickerdoodle Cookies

**48 COOKIES**

**PREP TIME:** 15 minutes / Cook time: 13 minutes

Who doesn't love snickerdoodles? These delightful cinnamon cookies satisfy sweet cravings and deliver the perfect blend of slightly crunchy on the outside and chewy on the inside. They're so easy to make, so I always make a double batch and freeze half. It's so great to scoop out some dough when you just *must* have a treat!

1½ cups (3 sticks) butter, at room temperature

1½ cups granulated sweetener, divided (see tip)

6 large eggs plus 1 additional yolk

½ cup heavy cream

1 tablespoon vanilla extract

1¼ cups coconut flour

2 teaspoons cinnamon, divided

1 teaspoon baking soda

1 teaspoon cream of tartar

½ teaspoon salt

1. Preheat the oven to 325°F. Line a baking sheet with parchment paper and set aside.

2. In a large mixing bowl, cream together the butter, 1 cup of sweetener, eggs and additional yolk, heavy cream, and vanilla.

3. In a small bowl, mix together the coconut flour, 1 teaspoon of cinnamon, baking soda, cream of tartar, and salt.

4. Gradually pour the flour mixture into the butter mixture and mix well.

5. In another small bowl, mix the remaining ½ cup of sweetener and the remaining 1 teaspoon of cinnamon.

6. Using a cookie scoop, drop a scoop of dough into your hand, roll it into a ball, and then roll the ball in the sweetener and cinnamon mixture. Place the dough ball on the prepared baking sheet and pat to flatten slightly. Repeat with the remaining cookie dough.

7. Bake for 13 minutes, turning the baking sheet halfway through the baking time. Let the cookies rest a few minutes before transferring to a wire rack.

**TIP:** For sweetener, I use Lakanto Monkfruit with Erythritol (Golden), but you can use whichever brand you like. Just try to pick one that is a 1:1 replacement for real sugar. If you like a crunchy cookie, increase the baking time to 15 minutes. A great addition is chopped macadamia nuts. Just be sure to add any additional carbs to your total.

---

**Per Serving (3 cookies)** Calories: 286; Total fat: 24g; Carbohydrates: 13g; Fiber: 8g; Protein: 5g; Sugar alcohols: 12g; Net carbs: 5g

# No-Bake Brownie Bites

**18 BROWNIE BITES**

**PREP TIME:** 15 minutes, plus 1 hour to chill

I owned a specialty cake shop for years and made a lot of cake balls. For me, the tastiest part was always the dough, especially right out of the freezer. These brownie bites are the closest thing I've made yet that satisfies that delicious memory. You should come out with approximately 18 brownie bites if you don't eat any dough.

4 tablespoons coconut flour

½ cup unsweetened baking cocoa powder

½ cup sugar-free confectioners' sugar

6 ounces cream cheese, at room temperature

2 tablespoons butter, at room temperature

3 tablespoons peanut butter

1 teaspoon vanilla extract

1 tablespoon water

¼ teaspoon salt

1. Line a baking sheet with parchment paper and set aside.

2. Put all the ingredients into a bowl and mix with your hands or a spatula. Really get it worked together until it has the consistency of play dough.

3. Place the bowl in the refrigerator for 30 minutes.

4. Using a cookie scoop, drop a scoop of dough into your hand, roll it into a ball, and place it on the prepared baking sheet. Repeat with the remaining dough.

5. Place the baking sheet in the freezer for 30 minutes. Once the brownie bites are frozen, store in a resealable bag or container in the refrigerator or freezer.

**TIP:** Possible add-ins include sugar-free chocolate chips, nuts, different flavored nut butters, and so much more. Get festive and roll them in sugar-free confectioners' sugar, finely chopped nuts, or sugar-free sprinkles. If your additions leave the dough too dry, add a little more water. Just be sure to add the additional carbs to your total.

---

**Per Serving (1 brownie bite)** Calories: 89; Total fat: 7g; Carbohydrates: 4.4g; Fiber: 2g; Protein: 2.3g; Sugar alcohols: 6.66g; Net carbs: 2.4g

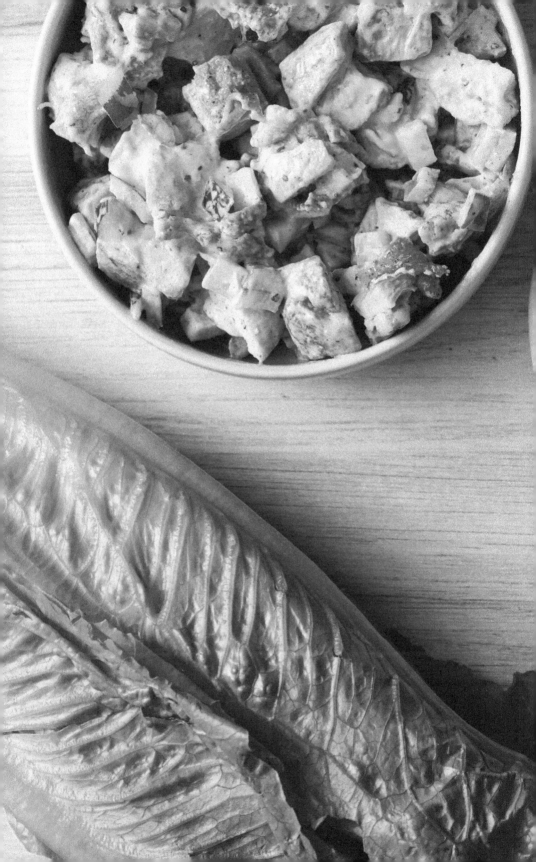

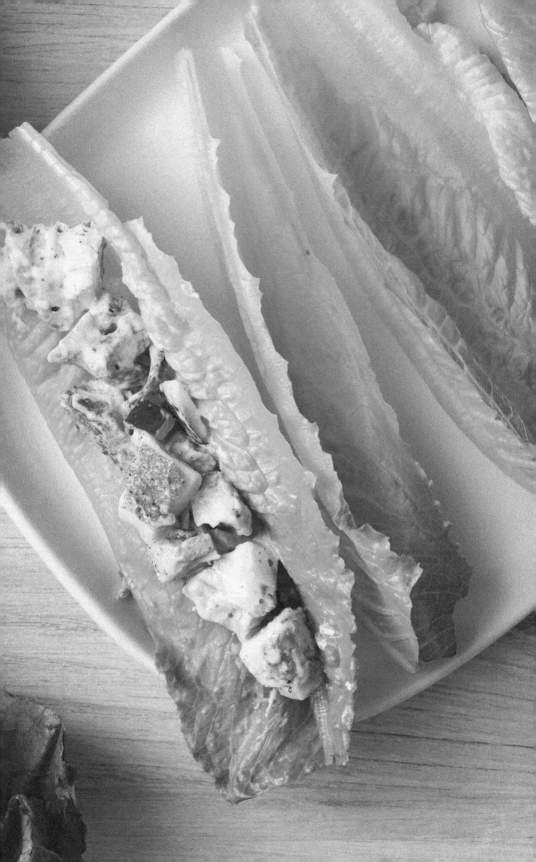

# Measurement Conversions

| | US STANDARD | US STANDARD (OUNCES) | METRIC (APPROXIMATE) |
|---|---|---|---|
| VOLUME EQUIVALENTS (LIQUID) | 2 tablespoons | 1 fl. oz. | 30 mL |
| | ¼ cup | 2 fl. oz. | 60 mL |
| | ½ cup | 4 fl. oz. | 120 mL |
| | 1 cup | 8 fl. oz. | 240 mL |
| | 1½ cups | 12 fl. oz. | 355 mL |
| | 2 cups or 1 pint | 16 fl. oz. | 475 mL |
| | 4 cups or 1 quart | 32 fl. oz. | 1 L |
| | 1 gallon | 128 fl. oz. | 4 L |
| VOLUME EQUIVALENTS (DRY) | ⅛ teaspoon | | 0.5 mL |
| | ¼ teaspoon | | 1 mL |
| | ½ teaspoon | | 2 mL |
| | ¾ teaspoon | | 4 mL |
| | 1 teaspoon | | 5 mL |
| | 1 tablespoon | | 15 mL |
| | ¼ cup | | 59 mL |
| | ⅓ cup | | 79 mL |
| | ½ cup | | 118 mL |
| | ⅔ cup | | 156 mL |
| | ¾ cup | | 177 mL |
| | 1 cup | | 235 mL |
| | 2 cups or 1 pint | | 475 mL |
| | 3 cups | | 700 mL |
| | 4 cups or 1 quart | | 1 L |
| | ½ gallon | | 2 L |
| | 1 gallon | | 4 L |
| WEIGHT EQUIVALENTS | ½ ounce | | 15 g |
| | 1 ounce | | 30 g |
| | 2 ounces | | 60 g |
| | 4 ounces | | 115 g |
| | 8 ounces | | 225 g |
| | 12 ounces | | 340 g |
| | 16 ounces or 1 pound | | 455 g |

|  | FAHRENHEIT (F) | CELSIUS (C) (APPROXIMATE) |
|---|---|---|
| OVEN TEMPERATURES | 250°F | 120°C |
|  | 300°F | 150°C |
|  | 325°F | 180°C |
|  | 375°F | 190°C |
|  | 400°F | 200°C |
|  | 425°F | 220°C |
|  | 450°F | 230°C |

# Resources

## MACRO CALCULATORS

My favorite macro calculator, from Maria Emmerich, is the one I use all the time: mariamindbodyhealth.com/keto-calculator.

Another macro calculator is from the great folks at Perfect Keto: perfectketo.com/keto-macro-calculator.

## WEBSITES

Below you'll find some resources that I have found invaluable on my journey.

www.charliefoundation.org
The Charlie Foundation for Ketogenic Therapies, founded in 1994, provides information about diet therapies for people with epilepsy, other neurological disorders, and select cancers. You will find so much information on their site.

www.perfectketo.com
Founded by Dr. Anthony Gustin, Perfect Keto focuses on improving health by providing products that help you reach your goals. I have used their MCT oil powder and collagen powder in my coffee every single morning since I started this lifestyle, and I love their snack bars, as well. Their website is a wealth of information with articles and recipes, and they also have a book titled *Keto Answers* to help newcomers to the keto journey.

www.mariamindbodyhealth.com
Maria Emmerich is a nutritionist who specializes in the ketogenic diet and exercise physiology. Her book *Keto* is a wealth of information, and she has written many cookbooks, as well.

www.cutdacarb.com
Cut Da Carb makes low-carb flatbreads, which have become a staple at our house. We make pizza, tortilla chips, and so much more with them.

www.gooddees.com

It's fun to bake goodies from scratch at home, but if you want to purchase some delicious low-carb baking mixes made with great ingredients, then Good Dee's is the place to go.

www.kettleandfire.com

Kettle and Fire makes some of the best bone broths and keto soups on the market.

www.keto-mojo.com

I have used ketone/glucose testing kits by Keto-Mojo for years and am a huge fan.

www.dropanfbomb.com

Another staple in our house, FBomb Nut Butters are some of the best high-fat snacks on the market.

www.scoutandcellar.com

Scout & Cellar is one of the best online wine clubs, selling organic, clean-crafted, naturally keto-friendly wine from boutique wineries around the world.

# References

## CHAPTER 1

Charlie Foundation for Ketogenic Therapies. "Keto for Epilepsy." Accessed November 25, 2019. https://charliefoundation.org /keto-for-epilepsy/.

Cleveland Clinic. "Study Looks at Ketogenic Diet to Treat PCOS and Infertility." Accessed November 25, 2019. https://consultqd .clevelandclinic.org/study-looks-at-ketogenic-diet -to-treat-pcos-and-infertility/.

Cooley, Jami. "Keto Diet: The Fat-Burning Health Benefits of Ketogenic Diet Foods." *University Health News*. December 19, 2018. https://universityhealthnews.com/daily/nutrition/keto-diet-health -benefits-of-ketogenic-diet/.

Holland, Kimberly. "How the Keto Diet May Help Fight Certain Cancer Tumors." *Healthline*. August 16, 2019. https://www.healthline .com/health-news/what-to-know-about-keto-diet-and-cancer.

Masood, Wajeed, and Kalyan R. Uppaluri. *Ketogenic Diet*. Treasure Island, FL: StatPearls Publishing, 2019. https://www.ncbi.nlm.nih.gov /books/NBK499830/.

MaxLove Project. "Metabolic Therapies in Cancer Treatment: A Research Summary." Accessed November 25, 2019. https://www .maxloveproject.org/ketogenic-research-summary.

Yancy, William S., Jr., Marjorie Foy, Allison M. Chalecki, Mary C. Vernon, and Eric C. Westman. "A Low-Carbohydrate, Ketogenic Diet to Treat Type 2 Diabetes." *Nutrition and Metabolism* 2, no. 34 (December 2005). doi:10.1186/1743-7075-2-34.

## CHAPTER 2

Arnarson, Atli. "8 Signs and Symptoms of Protein Deficiency." *Healthline*. October 31, 2017. https://www.healthline.com/nutrition /protein-deficiency-symptoms.

Blanton, Kayla. "'Keto Crotch' and 5 Other Scary Things That Could Happen to Your Body on the Keto Diet." *Insider*. February 28, 2019. https://www.insider.com/keto-diet-risks-body-2018-6#targetText=A%20 2007%20study%20on%20the,and%20a%20loss%20of%20electrolytes.

DiNicolantonio, James J., Sean C. Lucan, and James H. O'Keefe. "The Evidence for Saturated Fat and for Sugar Related to Coronary Heart Disease." *Progress in Cardiovascular Diseases* 58, no. 5 (March-April 2016): 464–72. doi:10.1016/j.pcad.2015.11.006.

Gupta, L., D. Khandelwal, S. Kalra, P. Gupta, D. Dutta, and S. Aggarwal. "Ketogenic Diet in Endocrine Disorders: Current Perspectives." *Journal of Postgraduate Medicine* 63, no. 4 (October-December 2017): 242–51. doi:10.4103/jpgm.JPGM_16_17.

Hooper, Lee, Nicole Martin, Asmaa Abdelhamid, and George Davey Smith. "Reduction in Saturated Fat Intake for Cardiovascular Disease." *Cochrane Database of Systematic Reviews* 2015, no. 6. doi:10.1002/14651858.CD011737.

Hyman, Mark. "The Secret Fat That Makes You Thin." *Dr.Hyman.com*. Accessed November 25, 2019. https://drhyman.com /blog/2016/02/04/the-secret-fat-that-makes-you-thin/.

Leonard, Jayne. "What Are the Signs of Ketosis?" *Medical News Today*. October 31, 2018. https://www.medicalnewstoday.com /articles/323544.php.

Nichols, Hannah. "Artery-Clogging Saturated Fat Myth Debunked." *Medical News Today*. April 26, 2017. https://www.medicalnewstoday .com/articles/317118.php.

Siri-Tarino, Patty W., Qi Sun, Frank B. Hu, and Ronald M. Krauss. "Meta-analysis of Prospective Cohort Studies Evaluating the Association of Saturated Fat with Cardiovascular Disease." *American Journal of Clinical Nutrition* 91, no. 3 (March 2010): 535–46. doi:10.3945 /ajcn.2009.27725.

St-Onge, M.P., and P.J. Jones. "Greater Rise in Fat Oxidation with Medium-Chain Triglyceride Consumption Relative to Long-Chain Triglyceride Is Associated with Lower Initial Body Weight and Greater Loss of Subcutaneous Adipose Tissue." *International Journal of Obesity* 27, no. 12 (December 2003): 1565–71. doi:10.1038/sj.ijo.0802467.

Tello, Monique. "Intermittent Fasting: Surprising Update." *Harvard Health Publishing*. June 29, 2018. https://www.health.harvard.edu /blog/intermittent-fasting-surprising-update-2018062914156.

# Index

# Acknowledgments

I would first of all like to thank my son Zack for all of his love, support, patience, and technical assistance regarding this book. I couldn't have done it without you. Also, my father, who has always backed me up, been on my side, and encouraged me to be the best I can be. A big thank you as well to Clara Song Lee and all the folks at Callisto Media who gave me a chance to "shine." And to David, my "Lovies," the love of my life. God surely saved the best for last when he led me to you.

# Author Biography

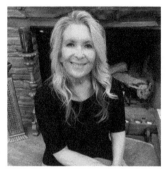 Mary Alexander is the author of the popular Instagram account @ketohabits, which she started in early 2016 for her own accountability. She decided something had to change with her health and weight, and on Valentine's Day 2016, she started the ketogenic lifestyle with her partner, David (referred to always as "Lovies"). Mary has lost 60-plus pounds with keto and still enjoys baking, as well as blogging and inspiring all those who follow her to learn how easy, effective, and life-changing keto can be. As the retired specialty cake owner of Mary Alexander Cakes, she brings a lot to the table as far as delicious recipes that have been ketofied. Her before-and-after keto accomplishments were featured in *Reader's Digest*.

Mary lives in Texas with Lovies, where they share three beautiful children, Zack, Kristina, and Chris. They enjoy family challenges and collectively have lost almost 200 pounds.

CPSIA information can be obtained
at www.ICGtesting.com
Printed in the USA
BVHW060718020920
587859BV00001B/1